COLOUR GU

PICTURE TE

CW00732006

Oral Medicine

David Wray MD BDS MB ChB FDS RCPS FDS RCS (Ed)

Associate Dean for Research and Professor of Oral Medicine
University of Glasgow Dental School
Honorary Consultant in Oral Medicine
Glasgow Dental Hospital and School NHS Trust
Glasgow, UK

John Gibson BDS MB ChB FDS (OM) RCPS FFD RCS (Irel)

Lecturer in Oral Medicine
University of Glasgow Dental School
Honorary Consultant in Oral Medicine
Glasgow Dental Hospital and School NHS Trust
Glasgow, UK

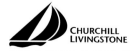

CHURCHILL
LIVINGSTONE

EDINBURGH   LONDON   NEW YORK   OXFORD   PHILADELPHIA
ST LOUIS   SYDNEY   TORONTO   1997

CHURCHILL LIVINGSTONE
An imprint of Elsevier Limited

© Pearson Professional Limited 1997
© Harcourt Publishers Limited 1999
© Elsevier Science Limited 2002. All rights reserved.
© Elsevier Limited 2003. All rights reserved.

First Edition 1997
 Reprinted 1999, 2002 (twice), 2003

ISBN 0-443-05301-4

British Library Cataloguing in Publication Data
A catalogue record for this book is available from the British Library

Library of Congress Cataloging in Publication Data
A catalog record for this book is available from the Library of Congress

For Churchill Livingstone
Publisher Michael Parkinson
Project manager Ninette Premdas
Project editor Jim Killgore
Project controller Kay Hunston
Design direction Erik Bigland

Medical knowledge is constantly changing. As new information
becomes available, changes in treatment, procedures, equipment
and the use of drugs become necessary. The authors and the
publishers have, as far as it is possible, taken care to ensure that
the information given in this text is accurate and up to date.
However, readers are strongly advised to confirm that the
information, especially with regard to drug usage, complies with
current legislation and standards of practice.

 ELSEVIER SCIENCE

your source for books,
journals and multimedia
in the health sciences

www.elsevierhealth.com

The
publisher's
policy is to use
paper manufactured
from sustainable forests

Printed in China

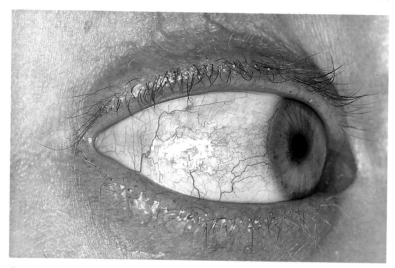

3. This patient complains of grittiness of her eyes.

a. What oral problems is she likely to complain of?
b. What may this syndrome be secondary to?

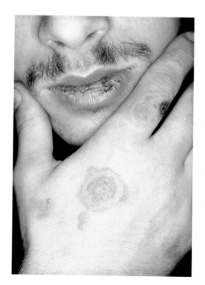

4.

a. What is the clinical diagnosis?
b. Is the lesion intra-epithelial or subepithelial?
c. Name a precipitating factor.

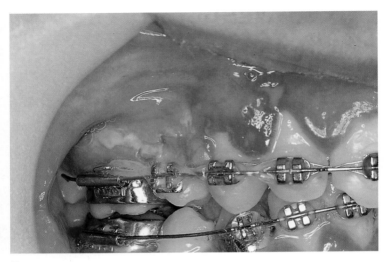

5. These lesions have been present for 4 days.

a. What is the most likely diagnosis?
b. Name two ways of confirming your diagnosis.

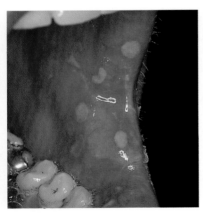

6. These lesions heal without scarring and are recurrent.

a. What is the diagnosis?
b. What parts of the mouth will be unaffected by these ulcers?
c. Are these ulcers more common in males or females?

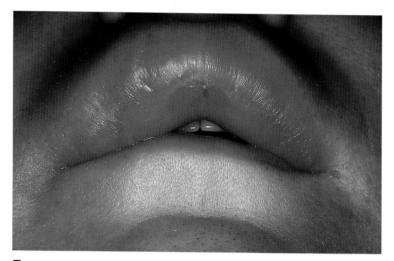

7. This boy presents with chronic lip swelling.

a. What is the clinical diagnosis?
b. What two systemic diseases may be associated with this condition?

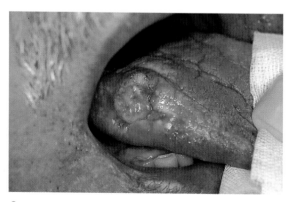

8. A 57-year-old man presented with this ulcer of 6 weeks duration.

a. What is the clinical diagnosis?
b. How would the diagnosis be established?
c. What may be relevant in the social history?
d. How may this lesion be treated?

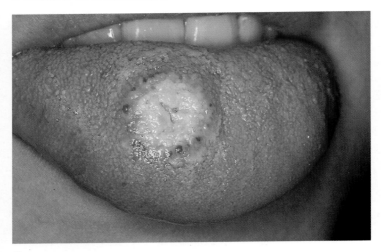

9. **This patient presents with a painless, well-circumscribed tongue ulcer of 10 days' duration.**

a. What differential diagnoses would you consider?
b. What are the appropriate investigations?

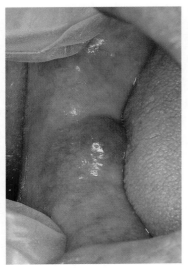

10. **This patient has noticed this lesion increasing in size over the last 2 years.**

a. What is the clinical diagnosis?
b. What is the most suitable treatment?
c. What complications may arise from this lesion?

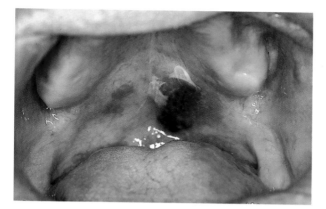

11. This patient presents with an intermittent history of blood-filled blisters restricted to the soft palate. These burst and heal without scarring within 10 days.

a. What is the diagnosis?
b. What are the immunofluorescent features?
c. What treatment should be prescribed?

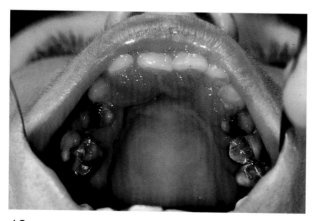

12. This woman who is 36 weeks pregnant presents with a gingival swelling.

a. What lesion does the photograph show?
b. What is the immediate management?
c. What is the prognosis?

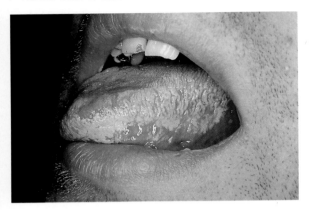

13. This 32-year-old man gives a 3 month history of malaise, fever and weight loss and has had two episodes of oral candidosis.

a. What is the clinical diagnosis?
b. What are the histological features?
c. How would you confirm the diagnosis?

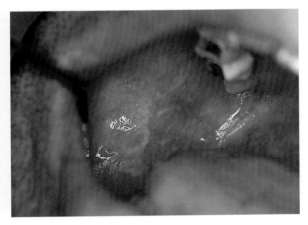

14. This 63-year-old man presents with asymptomatic white patches on his buccal mucosa.

a. What is the clinical diagnosis?
b. How would you confirm the diagnosis?
c. What treatment is required?

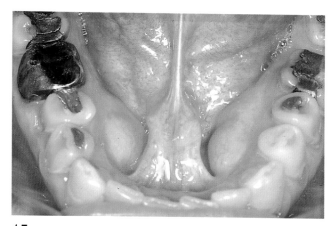

15. This 25-year-old man is concerned about the bilateral swellings of his mandible.

a. What is the diagnosis?
b. What is the prognosis?
c. What is the appropriate treatment?

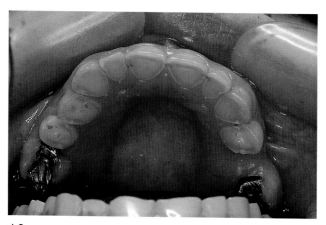

16. This 23-year-old woman is complaining that her teeth are becoming shorter.

a. What clinical lesions are seen?
b. What does the distribution of the lesions suggest about the aetiology?
c. How should she be managed?

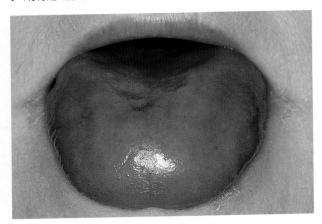

17. This 65-year-old woman presents with sensitivity of her tongue when drinking hot tea.

a. What is the clinical diagnosis?
b. What investigations would be appropriate?
c. What other oral lesions is she susceptible to?

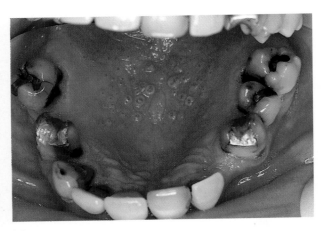

18. This 46-year-old man has attended for a routine dental appointment.

a. What is the lesion on his palate?
b. What is the cause?
c. How should he be managed?

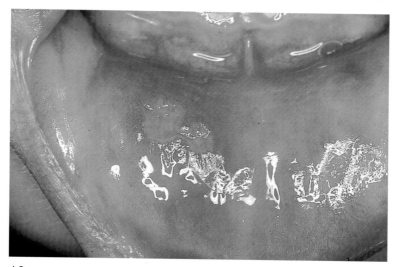

19. This patient presents with a history of a sore lip for 3 days and has had no previous similar episodes.

a. What is the diagnosis?
b. How would you manage the patient?

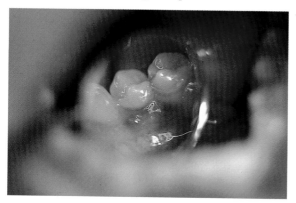

20. You notice this lesion during a routine dental examination.

a. What is the likely diagnosis?
b. How might you confirm this diagnosis?
c. How will you manage this patient?

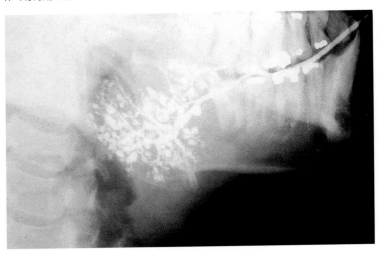

21. This patient has a long history of a dry mouth.

a. What investigation is shown in the photograph?
b. What features does the picture show?
c. In which patients would this investigation be contraindicated?

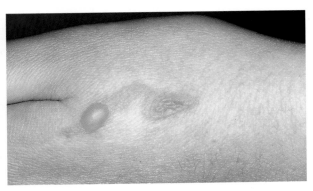

22. This woman has oral erosions in addition to her skin lesions.

a. What is the differential diagnosis?
b. What investigations are required to confirm the diagnosis?
c. What are the diagnostic features of these investigations?

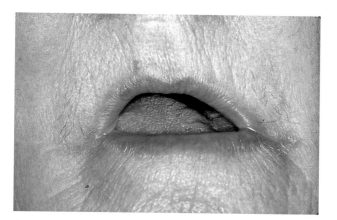

23. This 70-year-old edentulous woman is complaining of sores at the angles of her mouth.

a. What is the clinical diagnosis?
b. What factors might be important in the development of this condition?

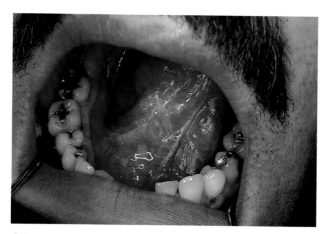

24. The above patient presents for routine dental examination and you notice a lesion on the floor of the mouth.

a. What external agents may contribute to this appearance?
b. What investigations should be carried out?

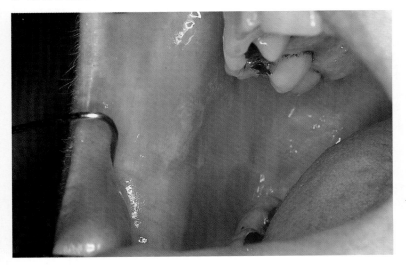

25. **In addition to these oral lesions, this patient has a facial rash which worsens in sunlight.**

a. What is the diagnosis?
b. What histological features might be evident?

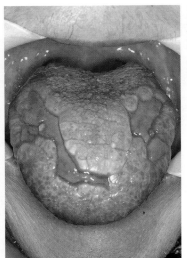

26. **This 60-year-old woman has long-standing erosive lichen planus.**

a. What are the histological features?
b. What are the chances of this lesion becoming malignant?

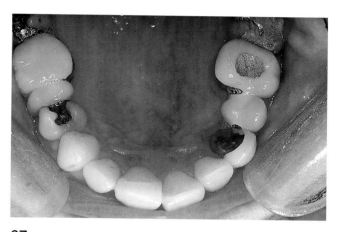

27. This patient was referred by her dentist for unexplained maxillary pain.

a. What is the diagnosis?
b. What is the appropriate treatment?

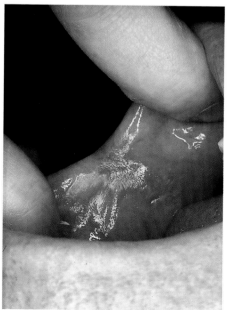

28. This patient presents with white patches on the inner aspect of the labial commissures.

a. What is the clinical diagnosis?
b. How would you confirm the diagnosis?
c. What external agent may be an aetiological cofactor?

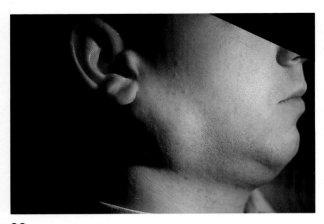

29. **The above patient presents with a right facial swelling which has been increasing in size over the last 3 years.**

a. What is the clinical diagnosis?
b. How would you confirm the diagnosis?
c. What is the appropriate treatment?

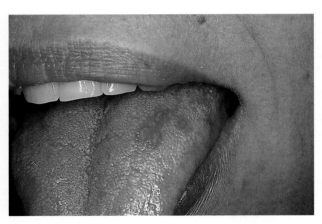

30. **This patient complains of ulcers on her tongue and buccal mucosa which occur every 2–3 weeks and last for 10 days.**

a. What is the clinical diagnosis?
b. What investigations are indicated?
c. How likely are these investigations to prove helpful?

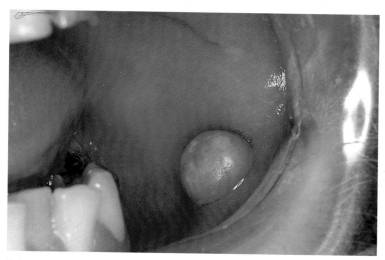

31. This 30-year-old man complains of a lump in his cheek which he has a tendency to bite.

a. What is the most likely diagnosis?
b. Is this lesion premalignant?
c. What is the appropriate treatment?

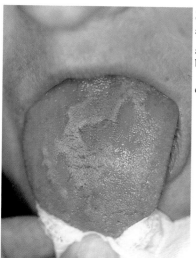

32. This patient has asymptomatic tongue lesions.

a. What is the diagnosis?
b. What skin disease may be associated with this appearance?
c. Are these lesions always restricted to the tongue?

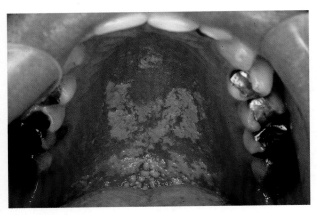

33. This 35-year-old man complains of roughness of his palate.

a. What is the clinical diagnosis?
b. What underlying causes should be considered?
c. How might you confirm the diagnosis at the chairside?

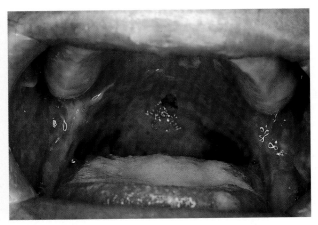

34. This 60-year-old woman has pemphigus vulgaris.

a. What type of disorder is pemphigus vulgaris?
b. What are the immunofluorescent features?
c. What is the usual treatment?

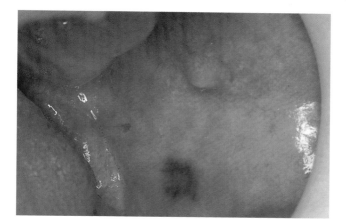

35. This patient complains of a brown lesion of increasing size which has been present for 3 months.

a. How would you diagnose this lesion?
b. What substance produces the brown coloration?

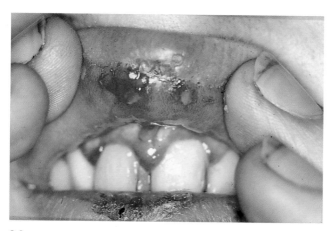

36. This 8-year-old boy has spontaneous bleeding from his gingivae.

a. What investigation would you carry out?
b. What other clinical features may be associated with this condition?

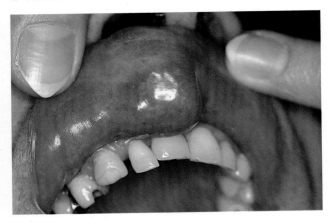

37. This 50-year-old woman presents with a 3 month history of a swelling of her upper lip. It was diagnosed by the referring practitioner as a mucocele.

a. What is the clinical diagnosis?
b. What is the appropriate treatment?

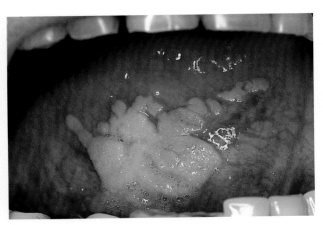

38. This young adult male has had a sublingual white patch for as long as he can remember.

a. What is the likely diagnosis?
b. How would you confirm this diagnosis?
c. What is the appropriate management of this lesion?

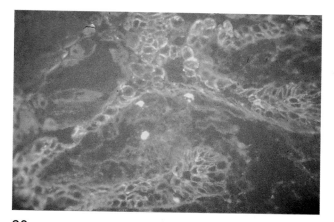

39. This is the immunofluorescent appearance of a biopsy from the buccal mucosa of a 55-year-old female.

a. Is this direct or indirect immunofluorescence?
b. What is the diagnosis in this patient?
c. Is she likely to have skin lesions?

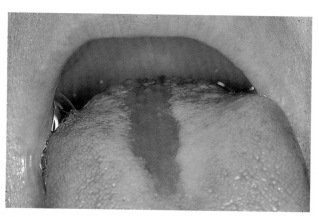

40. This 47-year-old asthmatic patient presents with an asymptomatic lesion on the dorsum of the tongue.

a. What is the clinical diagnosis?
b. What is a likely contributing factor in this patient's case?
c. What is the causative agent?

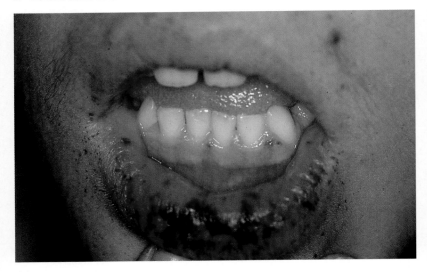

41. **This patient has had perioral freckles all her life.**

a. What systemic condition may this be associated with?
b. What investigation should be carried out?
c. What is the long-term prognosis?

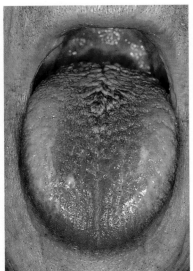

42. **This patient complains of a dirty tongue.**

a. What is the clinical diagnosis?
b. What may have caused this condition?
c. How would you treat it?

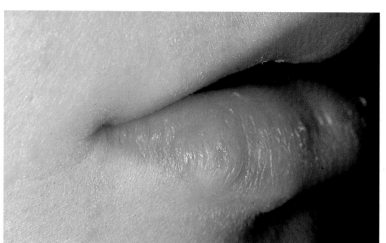

43. This 15-year-old female gets recurrent lesions on her lower lip.

a. What is the clinical diagnosis?
b. What is the causative agent?
c. How would you manage this patient?

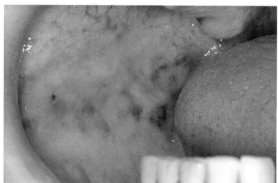

44. This Caucasian male has recently developed widespread intra-oral pigmentation.

a. Name two likely causes for this appearance.
b. How might you investigate the patient for systemic causes?

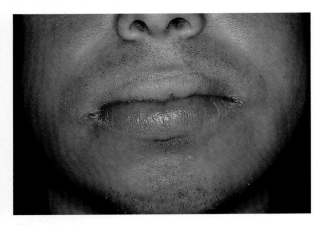

45. This 35-year-old male suffers from orofacial granulomatosis.

a. What investigations might be useful in excluding associated sarcoidosis?
b. What investigations may be valuable in excluding associated gut Crohn's disease?

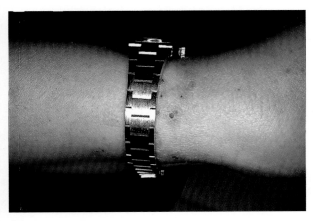

46. This 53-year-old woman has an itchy rash underneath her watch strap.

a. What is the likely diagnosis of the skin disorder?
b. What is this phenomenon called?
c. How common are oral problems in patients with this skin disease?

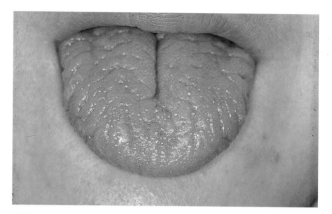

47. This patient experiences intermittent discomfort from his tongue.

a. What is the diagnosis?
b. What medical conditions may be associated with this appearance?
c. How should the patient be managed?

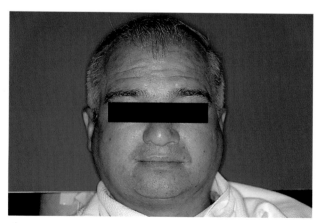

48. This patient presents with bilateral painless parotid gland swellings which have been present for 2 years.

a. What is the likely diagnosis?
b. What disorders may this condition be associated with?
c. What are the appearances on sialography?

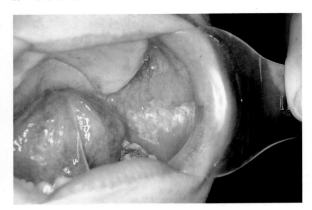

49. **This patient complains of tender white patches on the buccal mucosa.**

a. What is the clinical diagnosis?
b. Histologically, are there likely to be features of epithelial dysplasia?
c. Histologically, is there likely to be a dense submucosal inflammatory infiltrate?

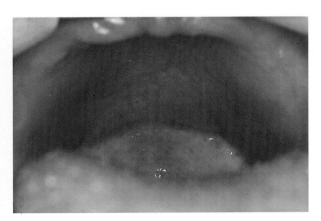

50. **This patient presents with a Newton's class II chronic erythematous candidosis.**

a. What is Newton's classification?
b. What topical agents are available to treat this condition?

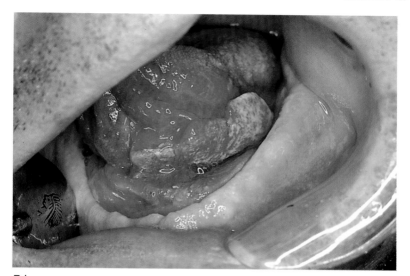

51. This 62-year-old patient presents with a painful ulcer of 4 months duration.

a. What is the clinical diagnosis?
b. How is this lesion likely to spread?

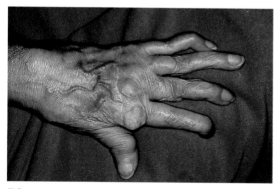

52. This 70-year-old woman has difficulty in attending for dental treatment due to her arthritis.

a. What is the diagnosis?
b. Name three clinical signs shown in the photograph.

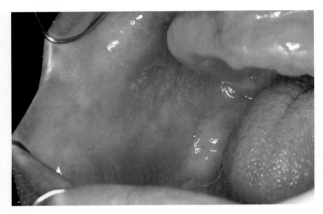

53. **This patient has asymptomatic yellow spots in the buccal mucosa.**

a. What is the diagnosis?
b. What is the nature of these spots?
c. What treatment is required?

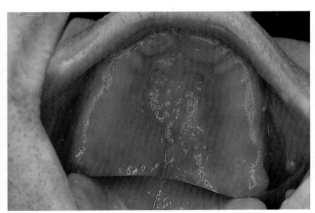

54. **This patient complains of tenderness under the upper denture.**

a. What is the clinical diagnosis?
b. What is the relevance of the denture to this condition?
c. What is the likely infecting agent?

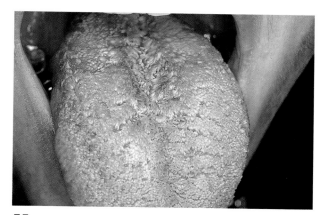

55. This patient complains of dryness of the mouth which has been getting worse over the last year.

a. What are the most common causes of a dry mouth?
b. What are the common oral complications of xerostomia?

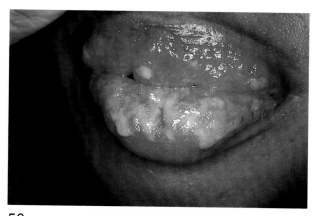

56. This patient complains of a sore mouth and crusting of the lips of 1 week duration.

a. What is the most likely diagnosis?
b. How would you confirm this diagnosis?
c. What is the appropriate treatment?

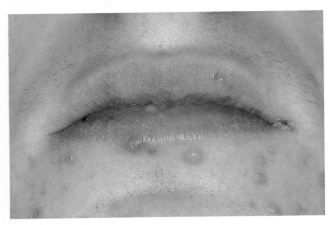

57. **This patient complains of oral soreness and lymphadenopathy of 2 days duration.**

a. What is the likely diagnosis?
b. Why is this not, clinically, recurrent aphthous stomatitis?
c. What is the appropriate treatment?

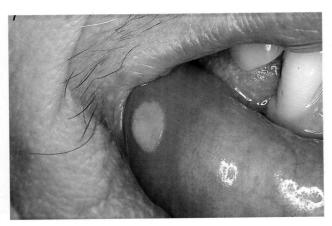

58. **This patient suffers from recurrent oral ulceration.**

a. Is there a genetic component to these ulcers?
b. This patient is an ex-smoker. Is this relevant?

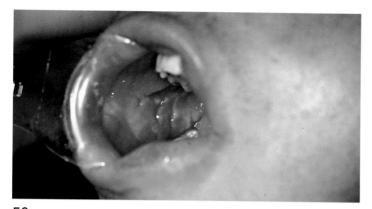

59. This patient also has a fissured tongue and a history of facial nerve palsies.

a. What is the clinical diagnosis?
b. What causes the facial nerve palsy?

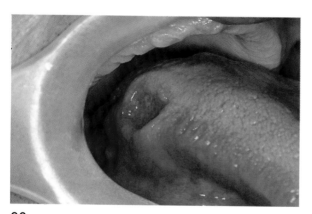

60. This 60-year-old woman has a 3 month history of this oral lesion which, histologically, is a carcinoma.

a. What is the relationship between her smoking and drinking habits and this lesion?
b. What specialist treatment would you explain to her that she is likely to receive?
c. What clinical examination would you undertake?

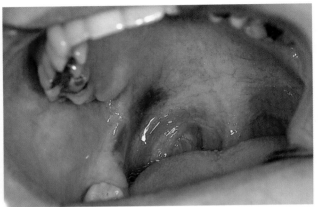

61. This patient developed submucosal haemorrhage after a local anaesthetic injection.

a. What blood tests would you consider appropriate?
b. If the patient were on warfarin, what pre-operative measures would be required before an extraction?

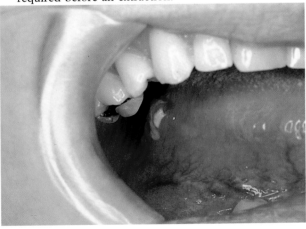

62. This patient presented complaining of a painful side to the tongue.

a. What is the likely diagnosis?
b. How would you investigate this patient?
c. How would you treat this patient?

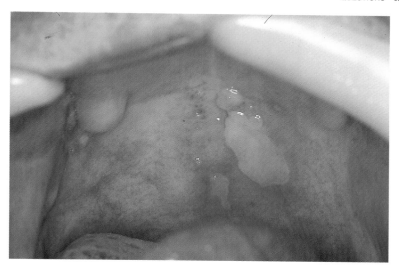

63. This patient has developed blisters which turn into ulcers and fail to heal.

a. What is the likely diagnosis?
b. What are the immunofluorescent features?
c. What is the appropriate treatment?

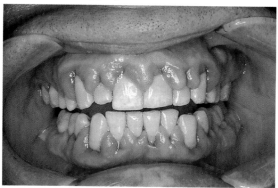

64. This patient has chronic overgrowth of the gingivae.

a. What drugs may be responsible for this appearance?
b. How would you manage this patient?

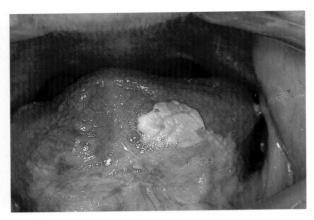

65. **This patient is asymptomatic but you note this appearance on the floor of the mouth.**

a. What is the clinical diagnosis?
b. What questions would you ask the patient?
c. What investigations would you carry out in the first instance?

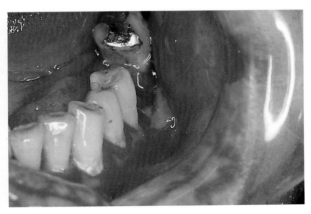

66. **This patient complains of tenderness in the mouth on eating hot or spicy foods.**

a. What is the clinical diagnosis?
b. What precipitating factors may there be?
c. What is the mainstay of treatment in this patient?

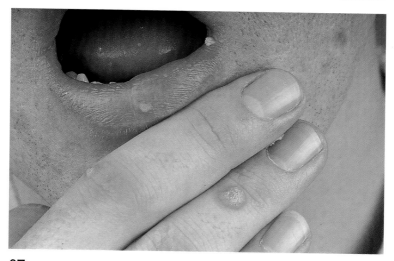

67. This young man complained of white lumps on his lower lip.

a. What is the diagnosis?
b. What is the causative agent?
c. What is the treatment?

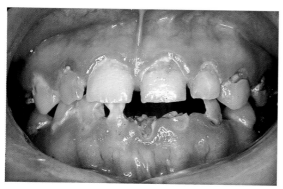

68. This patient has had radiotherapy for a malignancy.

a. What is the clinical problem?
b. How might further deterioration be prevented?
c. How should the patient be managed?

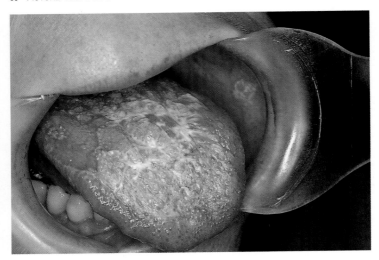

69. This 55-year-old woman has had long-standing reticular lichen planus which is asymptomatic.

a. What therapy does she require?
b. What nail changes may be associated with lichen planus?

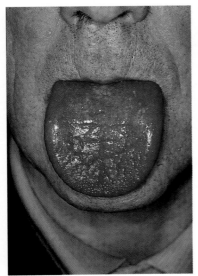

70. This 65-year-old man complains of a sensitive tongue and extreme difficulty in swallowing.

a. What may be the cause of his dysphagia.
b. What may be the underlying cause?
c. What complication may arise in this condition?

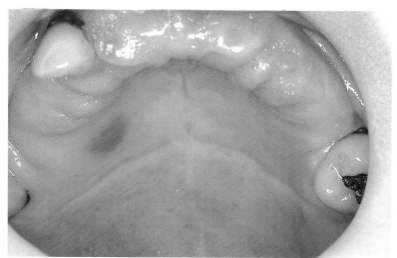

71. This patient's dentist has noticed a brown lesion in the patient's mouth on routine clinical examination.

a. What is the most likely diagnosis?
b. What is the appropriate investigation for this patient?

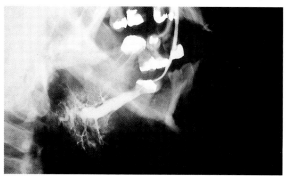

72. This patient complains of intermittent swelling of the right parotid gland.

a. What does this sialogram show?
b. How should this patient be treated?

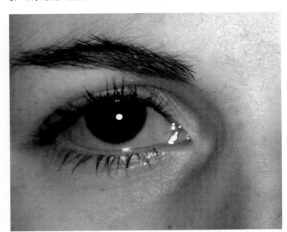

73. This young girl has a dental anomaly.

a. What generalised disease does she suffer from?
b. What is the dental anomaly she suffers from?

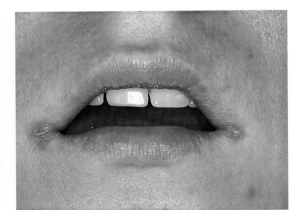

74. This young boy is complaining of sores at the corners of his mouth.

a. What is the clinical diagnosis?
b. What are the most likely infective agents?
c. How should this boy be managed?

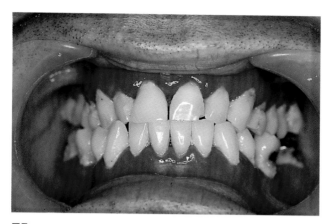

75. This patient developed sore, inflamed gums 10 days previously.

a. What is the clinical diagnosis?
b. What conditions may have caused this appearance?
c. How should this patient be managed?

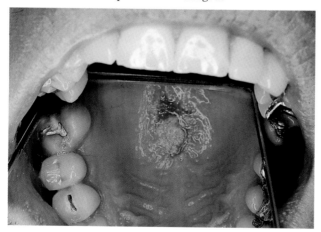

76. This patient presents with a long history of ulceration and discomfort of the palate.

a. What is the clinical diagnosis?
b. How could you confirm this diagnosis?
c. What blood tests would it be important to carry out?

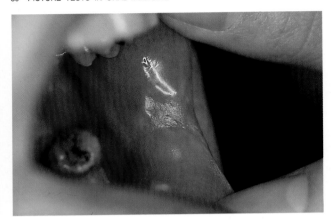

77. **This patient presents with white patches bilaterally inside the angles of his mouth.**

a. What is the clinical diagnosis?
b. What investigations are necessary in this patient?
c. What is the appropriate treatment?

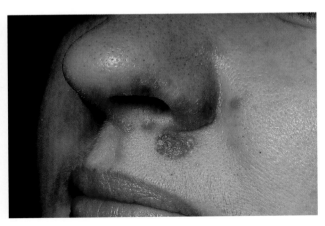

78. **This patient presents with a severe pain on one side of the face associated with blistering of the skin.**

a. What is the diagnosis?
b. How could you confirm the diagnosis?
c. When will this patient's pain resolve?

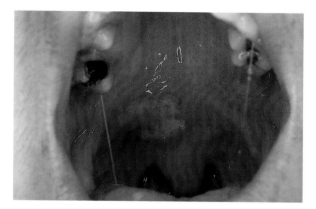

79. This patient has a history of recurrent oral ulceration. This ulcer has been present for 5 weeks.

a. What is the clinical diagnosis?
b. What investigations should be carried out?
c. What immediate management of this patient is indicated?

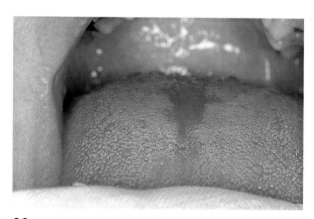

80. This patient is asymptomatic but you notice a smooth red patch on the dorsum of the tongue.

a. What is the likely diagnosis?
b. How could you confirm this diagnosis?
c. What may be the precipitating factor in this condition?
d. What is the appropriate treatment?

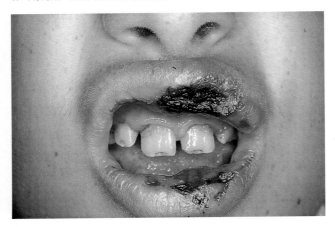

81. This child is being treated for acute lymphocytic leukaemia. You are asked to advise on his oral condition.

a. What therapies would you recommend for this child?
b. How would you treat a painful carious premolar in this child?

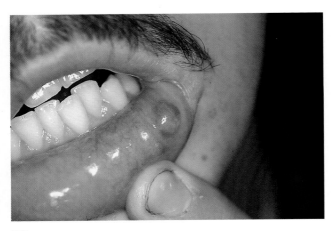

82. This lower lip swelling has recurred three times in the last year.

a. What is the clinical diagnosis?
b. What is the treatment of this condition?
c. What may the histology show?

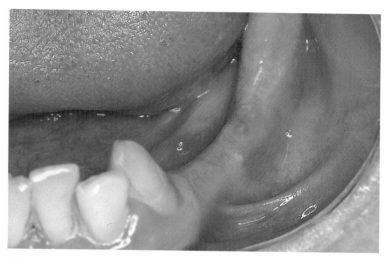

83. This area of pigmentation was found on routine examination and was causing the patient significant anxiety.

a. What caused the pigmentation?
b. How could you confirm this simply?

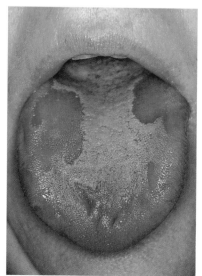

84. This patient is concerned by the appearance of, and discomfort from, her tongue.

a. What is the diagnosis?
b. Are there any known associations with other medical conditions?
c. How should the patient be managed?

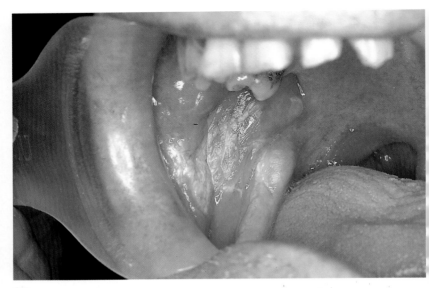

85. This patient is asymptomatic but you notice this appearance on the inside of the buccal mucosa.

a. What is the clinical diagnosis?
b. How would you manage this condition?

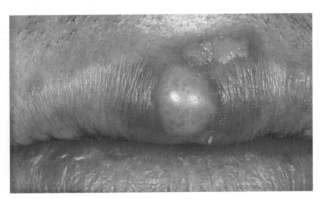

86. This young man gets recurrent herpetic lesions on his upper lip.

a. What is the pathogenesis of this lesion?
b. What precipitating factors are known for herpes labialis?

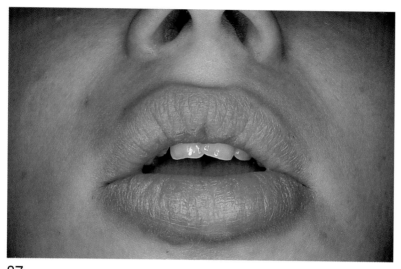

87. This patient is suffering from orofacial granulomatosis.

a. What are the other oral manifestations apart from lip swelling?

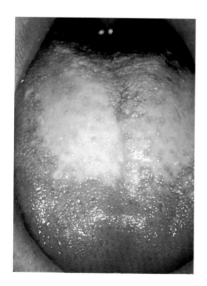

88. This tongue lesion is associated with similar lesions on the left and right buccal mucosa.

a. What is the clinical diagnosis?
b. What generalised disease processes may be associated with this lesion?

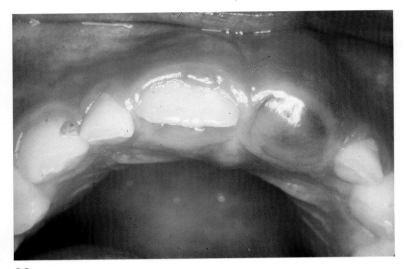

89. **This painful swelling occurred in a 6-year-old boy.**

a. What is the clinical diagnosis?
b. How would you treat this lesion?
c. What would be the histological features if a portion of this lesion were excised?

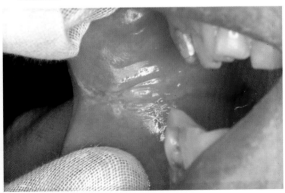

90. **This patient has a similar appearance on both commissures.**

a. What is the clinical diagnosis?
b. What special stains would you use histologically?

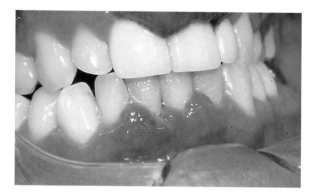

91. This 22-year-old man has been complaining of malaise and swollen glands for the last 10 days.

a. What condition is it important to exclude from the differential diagnosis?
b. What should your initial screening test be?
c. What oral problems are likely if the diagnosis is confirmed?

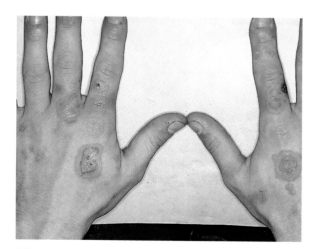

92. This lesion appeared in an individual with a history of recurrent stomatitis.

a. What are these lesions?
b. What is the most likely clinical diagnosis?

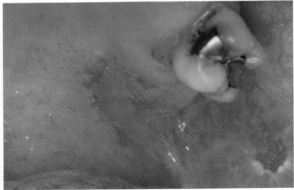

93. **This 46-year-old woman has had this palatal lesion for the last 2½ months.**

a. What is the clinical diagnosis?
b. How may this condition be subdivided?
c. What is the treatment of this lesion?

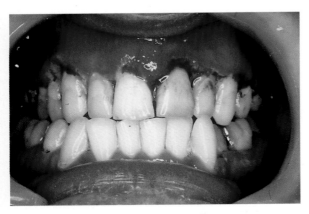

94. **This patient presents with a history of spontaneous gingival bleeding and halitosis.**

a. What is the clinical diagnosis?
b. What are the clinical symptoms and signs?
c. What organisms are involved?
d. What generalised diseases might be involved?

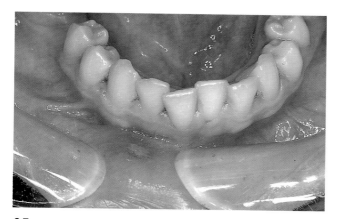

95. This 15-year-old boy has had several attacks of oral ulceration and gingivitis at approximately 3-weekly intervals.

a. What is the clinical diagnosis?
b. What further tests are required?
c. What is the basic defect involved?

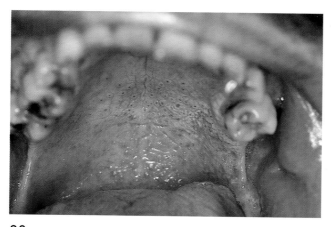

96. This patient's palatal appearance was noticed on routine examination.

a. What is the clinical diagnosis?
b. What other oral lesions should you look for?

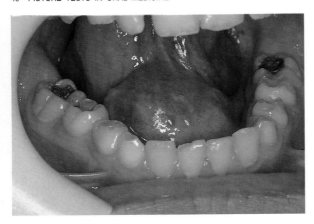

97. **This young adult presented with an intermittent swelling of the floor of the mouth.**

a. What is the clinical diagnosis?
b. What is the most common cause?
c. What is the best treatment?

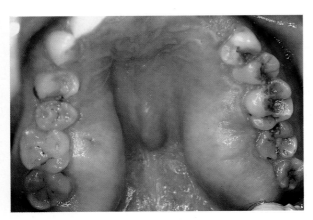

98. **This patient presents with a hard bony lump on the roof of the mouth and enlarged tuberosities.**

a. What is the palatal swelling?
b. What other conditions may this be associated with?

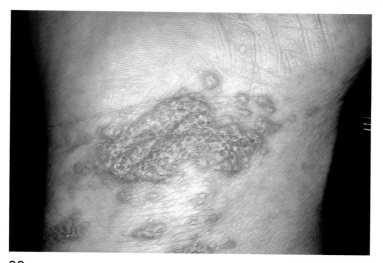

99. This woman presented with an itchy rash on her forearm and oral lesions.

a. What is the clinical diagnosis?
b. How many people have oral lesions and skin lesions together?
c. What is the natural history of these skin lesions?

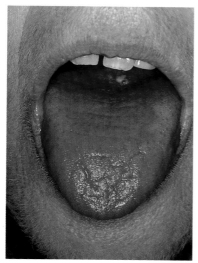

100. This patient has Crohn's disease and underwent gastrointestinal surgery 12 years previously.

a. What haematinic deficiency is she likely to have?
b. How should she be managed?

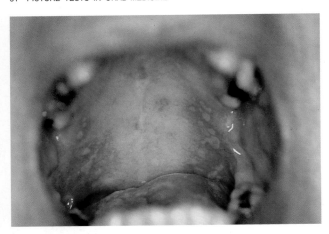

101. This young boy presented with severe painful ulceration, restricted to the soft palate, which had not occurred previously.

a. What is the clinical diagnosis?
b. What is the causative agent?
c. What other condition involving oral symptoms is caused by a similar agent?

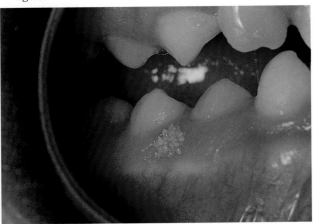

102. This warty lesion appeared on the gingival margin of a 12-year-old child.

a. What is the likely pathogenesis of this lesion?
b. What is the most appropriate treatment?

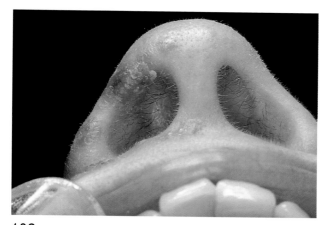

103. This woman presents with right-sided palatal ulceration and these skin lesions.

a. What is the clinical diagnosis?
b. What may be a long-term complication of this condition?

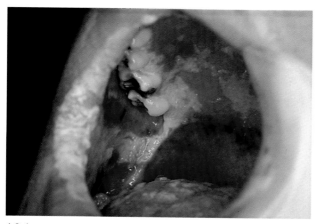

104. This boy with hypoadrenocorticism has had long-standing oral problems.

a. What two conditions are seen in the mouth?
b. What is the aetiology of the pigmented lesions?
c. What is the management of the white lesions?

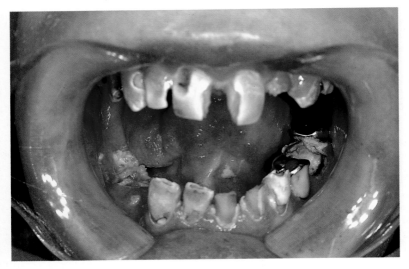

105. **This patient has undergone radiotherapy to the head and neck for malignancy.**

a. What changes have occurred as a result of this treatment?
b. What is the pathogenesis of this problem?

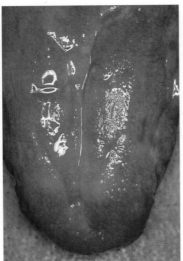

106. **This patient was 'lost to follow-up' by the general surgeons who removed his ileum some years previously.**

a. What was his likely gastrointestinal disease?
b. What is wrong with his mouth?
c. What is the appropriate management?

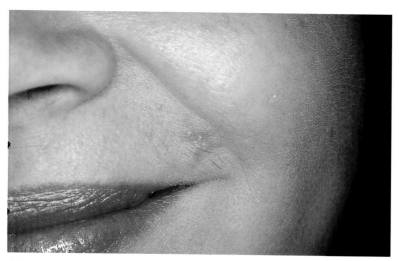

107. This 30-year-old woman presented with this skin lesion 4 days after dental treatment.

a. What is the likely diagnosis?
b. What is a more usual site for this lesion?

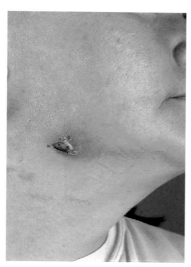

108. This patient presented with a discharging sinus over the mandible.

a. What is the pathogenesis of this lesion?
b. What unusual organism could be involved?
c. What would be the appropriate treatment?

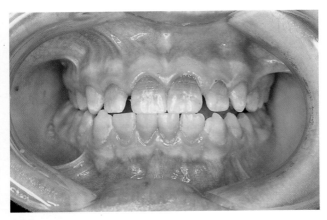

109. **This patient has a history of cystic fibrosis.**

a. What dental abnormality is seen?
b. Between what ages did the interference with development occur?
c. How could this abnormality be managed?

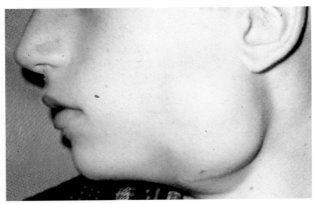

110. **This patient has osteomas and soft tissue tumours. Other family members are affected.**

a. What is the diagnosis?
b. What is the inheritance pattern of this disorder?
c. What gastrointestinal lesions occur in this disorder?
d. Is there a risk of malignant transformation in this disorder?

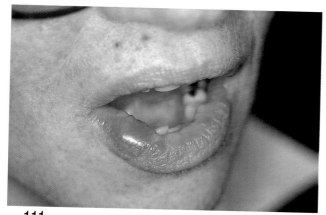

111. This young man developed a lip swelling 5 minutes after having a temporary crown inserted.

a. What is the clinical diagnosis?
b. What is the likely cause?
c. What is the immediate treatment?

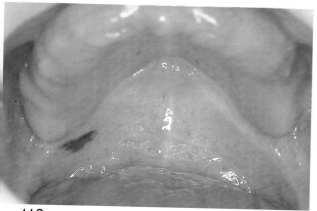

112. This area of pigmentation was found on routine examination.

a. List the differential diagnosis of a pigmented lesion.
b. How should the patient be managed?

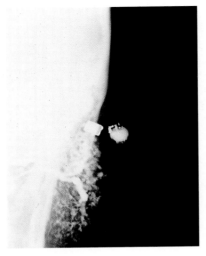

113. This radiograph demonstrates the features of a condition which often has very obvious oral manifestations.

a. Describe the radiographic features and name the condition.
b. What oral features might be evident on examination of the patient?

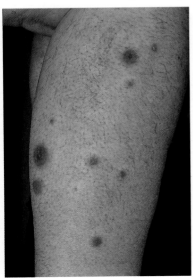

114. This patient had severe oral and lip bullae in association with these skin lesions.

a. What condition does the patient have?
b. What predisposing factors are recognised?

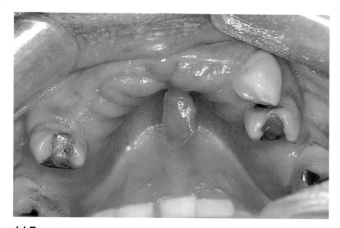

115. This lesion is seen in a 46-year-old patient requesting new dentures.

a. What is the diagnosis?
b. What is the aetiology?
c. What treatment should be carried out?

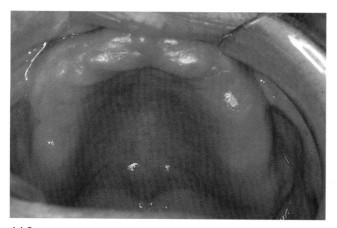

116. This patient has attended for new dentures.

a. What is the diagnosis?
b. What investigations are appropriate for this patient?
c. What non-drug measures should be instituted?

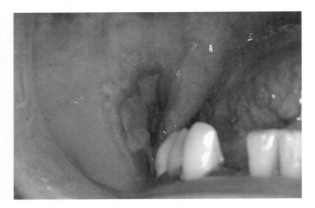

117. **This patient with rheumatoid arthritis has a unilateral erosion on her buccal mucosa which has been present for several months.**

a. What is the clinical diagnosis?
b. What is the most likely aetiological agent?
c. What is the appropriate management of this case?

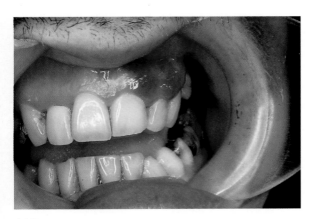

118. **This 26-year-old male presented with a bluish swelling of his gingival margin.**

a. What is the most likely clinical diagnosis?
b. What concurrent condition may he be suffering from?
c. How could this lesion be managed?

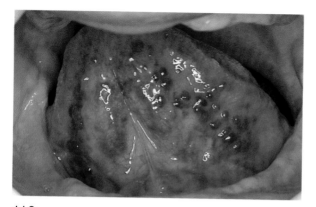

119. This 65-year-old woman was concerned about the possibility of oral cancer because of the appearance under her tongue.

a. What is the clinical diagnosis?
b. What is the appropriate management?

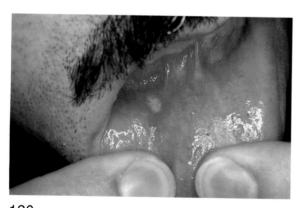

120. This 33-year-old patient had a repeatedly low vitamin B$_{12}$ level on haematological examination.

a. What peripheral blood changes may be seen in association with this B$_{12}$ deficiency?
b. What are the causes of B$_{12}$ deficiency?
c. What investigations would be appropriate in determining the cause of the B$_{12}$ deficiency?

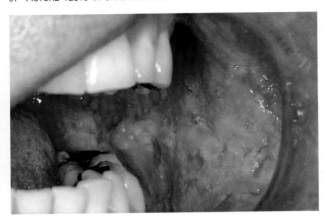

121. This patient has a history of ulcerative colitis and has developed a foul-smelling stomatitis.

a. What is the clinical diagnosis?
b. What are the histological features?
c. What is the appropriate management?

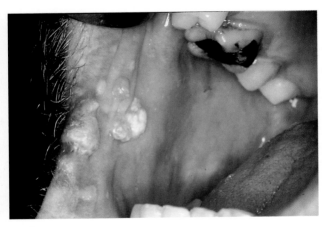

122. This 35-year-old male presents with a warty growth at the corner of his mouth.

a. What is the clinical diagnosis?
b. What systemic factors may be involved?
c. What is the management of this lesion?

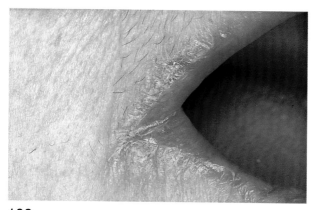

123. This 83-year-old woman has persistent angular cheilitis despite repeated antifungal therapy.

a. What organisms, apart from *Candida*, may be involved?
b. What systemic factors may be involved?

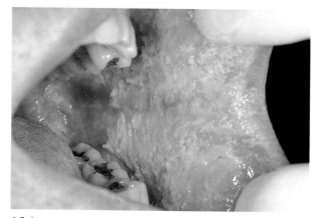

124. This patient has a long-standing white appearance of the oral mucosa. Other members of the family are also affected.

a. What is the diagnosis?
b. How would you confirm the diagnosis?
c. What histological features might be evident?

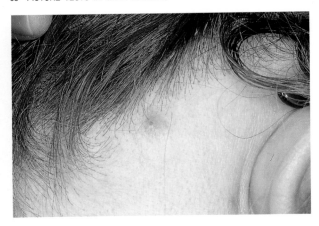

125. **This patient has pustular lesions on her skin which arise as a result of minor trauma. She also has oral ulceration.**

a. What other questions would it be important to ask this patient?
b. How could you predict the chances of eye involvement in this patient?
c. How may the eyes be affected?

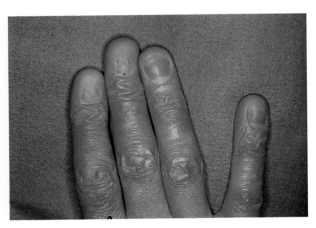

126. **This 28-year-old male has epidermolysis bullosa.**

a. What oral problems may he have?
b. What precautions would you take when carrying out routine dental treatment?

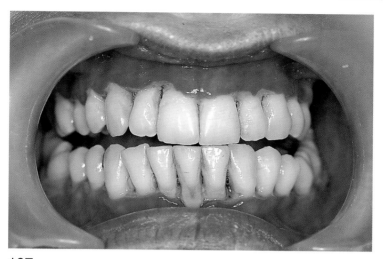

127. This patient, who is known to be HIV-seropositive, presents with rapidly progressing periodontal problems.

a. What additional cross-infection procedures are appropriate in this patient?
b. Is antibiotic prophylaxis necessary to work on this patient?
c. What is the appropriate management of the periodontal condition?

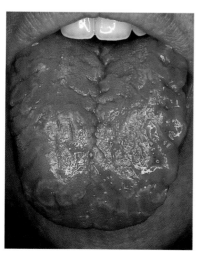

128. This patient presents for routine dental examination and her tongue is noticed to have this appearance.

a What is the clinical diagnosis?
b. What is the significance of the fissuring?
c. What is the prognosis of this condition?

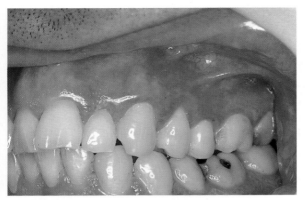

129. This patient presents with a recent onset of inflammation of gingivae, particularly in the buccal regions.

a. What is the clinical entity?
b. What may have produced such a lesion?
c. What is the immediate treatment of this patient?
d. If the condition fails to resolve, how would you manage this patient?

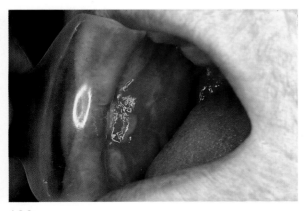

130. This patient with known lichen planus presents with a blister on her buccal mucosa.

a. What type of lichen planus is this?
b. What is the mechanism responsible for the blister arising?

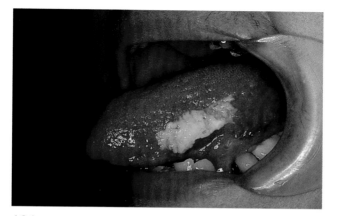

131. This 45-year-old woman presented complaining of a recent white patch appearing on the side of her tongue.

a. What is the clinical diagnosis?
b. What is the particular treatment in this patient's case?
c. What is the long-term follow-up of this patient?

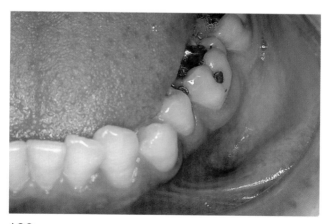

132. This area of pigmentation was alarming for a female patient who had recently read about 'oral cancer' in a magazine.

a. How should this patient be managed?
b. What is the most common intra-oral site for malignant melanoma?

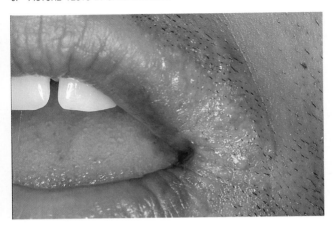

133. This lip lesion recurs frequently in a 24-year-old student, especially around examination times.

a. What is the diagnosis?
b. Are further investigations required?

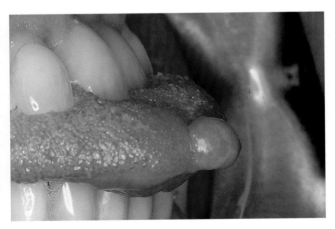

134. This appearance was found in a patient with an inadequate partial upper denture.

a. What is the diagnosis?
b. Why has the lesion appeared at this site?

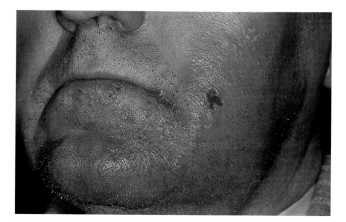

135. This 58-year-old man developed a burning discomfort on the left side of his mandible and face.

a. What is the diagnosis?
b. What is the necessary treatment?

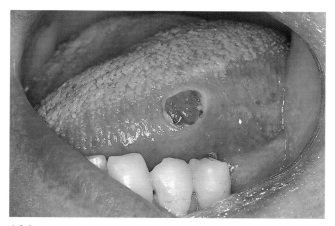

136. This 60-year-old woman presented in a very agitated state, fearful that this recent lesion was oral cancer.

a. What is the likely diagnosis?
b. What are the histological features?
c. What management would be required?

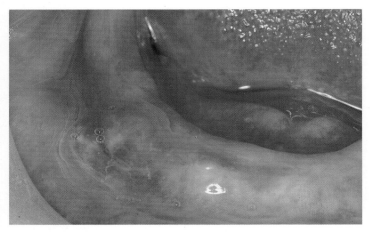

137. This 48-year-old edentulous male attended for the provision of new dentures. This lesion was found by the examining dentist.

a. What is the likely diagnosis?
b. The patient had experienced intermittent paraesthesia of his lower lip. What is the explanation for this?

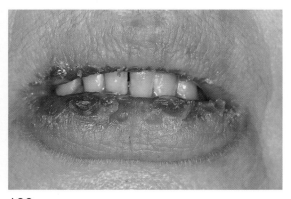

138. A 50-year-old woman presented with lip and oral lesions following a severe respiratory tract infection.

a. What is the likely diagnosis?
b. What is the likely precipitant, in view of the history?

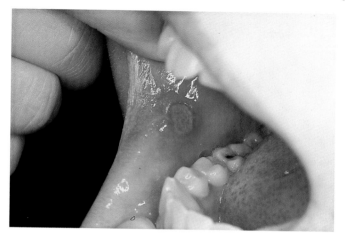

139. This patient has recurrent mouth ulcers.

a. What topical medications might be helpful?

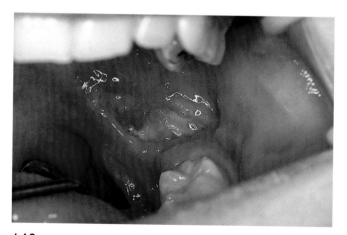

140. This patient has an underlying gastrointestinal disease.

a. What is it likely to be?
b. Why is oral mucosal cobblestoning a feature?

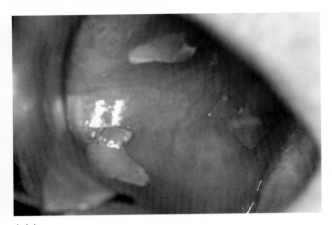

141. A 63-year-old female patient presents with a history of blood-filled blisters affecting the oral mucosa. This is the mucosal picture on examination.

a. What is the likely diagnosis?
b. What other oral manifestations are possible?
c. What treatment options should be considered?

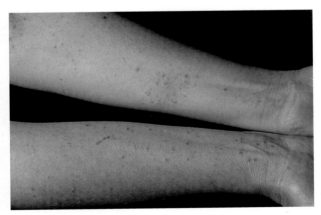

142. This patient has associated oral lesions.

a. What is the likely diagnosis?
b. What variants of the oral lesions are possible?

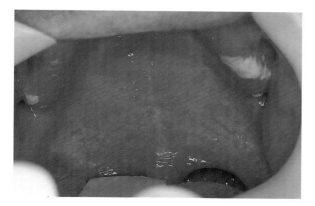

143. These white patches scrape off to reveal a raw, bleeding mucosal surface.

a. What is the diagnosis?
b. What systemic factors could have predisposed to this?
c. What local causes should be considered?

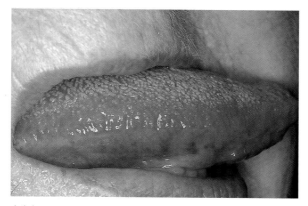

144. This 48-year-old woman developed a burning discomfort of her tongue 6 months previously, following the death of her husband.

a. What is the likely diagnosis in this patient?
b. What investigations should be performed routinely on such patients?
c. How should this patient be managed?

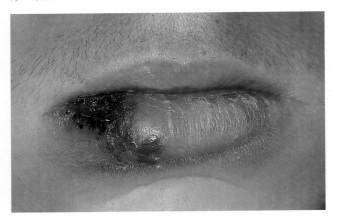

145. This 12-year-old boy returns to your surgery in great pain following dental treatment under local anaesthesia the previous day.

a. What is the likely cause of this lesion?
b. What treatment is appropriate?

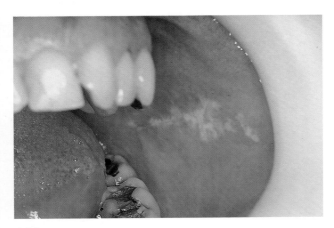

146. This is the appearance inside the mouth of an anxious 25-year-old school teacher, complaining of facial pain.

a. What is the likely cause of this appearance?
b. How might the patient be managed?

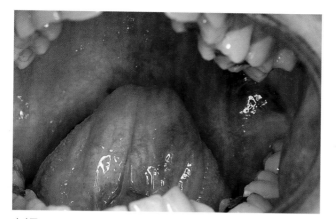

147. This 25-year-old man comes to your surgery for routine dental care, having just arrived from abroad.

a. What is the likely diagnosis?
b. What are the management considerations?

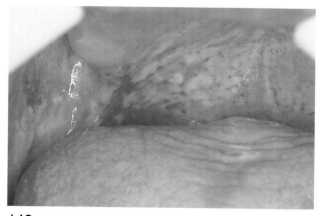

148. This lesion is found on the palate of a 48-year-old male smoker.

a. What is the clinical diagnosis?
b. What factors are important in the aetiology of this lesion?
c. How should the patient be managed?

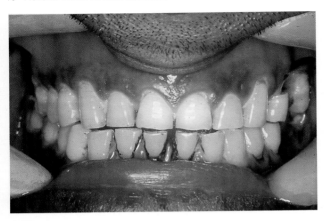

149. **This appearance was evident in a 28-year-old Asian patient.**

a. How concerned would you be about the very obvious areas of oral pigmentation?

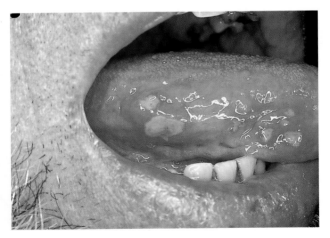

150. **These aphthous ulcers may be associated with systemic diseases.**

a. Which gastrointestinal diseases have been linked with aphthae?
b. Which immunological diseases have been linked with aphthae?

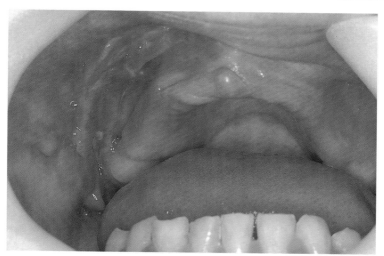

151. This lesion in the sulcus was observed in a long-term wearer of dentures.

a. What is the diagnosis?
b. What causes this problem?
c. How should the lesion be treated?

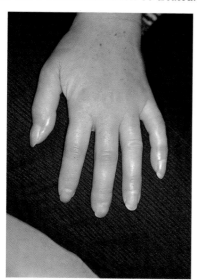

152. The above patient complains of a dry mouth.

a. What condition does her hand show?
b. What oral condition is she suffering from?

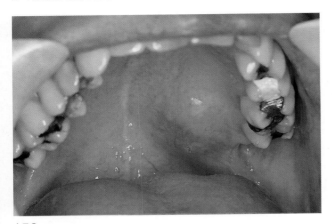

153. This palatal swelling was reported by the patient to have been present for some years.

a. What is the likely diagnosis?
b. How should the patient be managed?
c. What histological features would confirm the diagnosis?

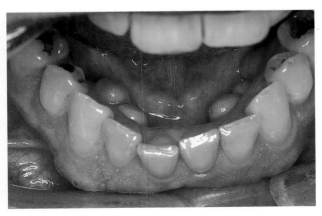

154. These multiple lumps were noticed at routine examination in a patient who thought they were 'normal'.

a. What is the likely diagnosis?
b. How should the patient be managed?
c. What difficulties could arise for future dental treatment?

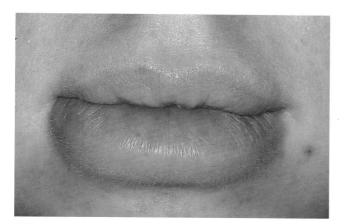

155. This teenage patient has a chronically swollen lip, with no other symptoms or signs.

a. What differential diagnoses should be considered?

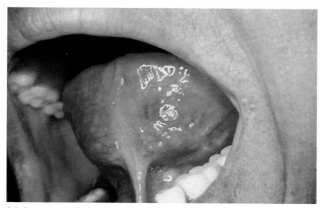

156. This lesion was causing problems for the patient and preventing adequate oral hygiene.

a. What is the diagnosis?
b. How should it be managed?

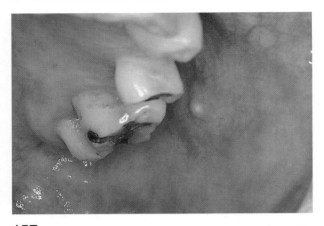

157. This young man complained of a hard swelling in his left buccal mucosa.

a. What is the clinical diagnosis?
b. What is the immediate management?

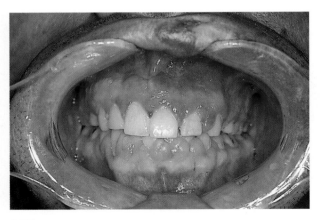

158. The patient with this clinical appearance also suffers from epilepsy.

a. What is the likely diagnosis?
b. There is an obvious clue to the patient's current seizure control drug. What is the clinical sign and what is the drug?
c. How might dental treatment be influenced in this patient?

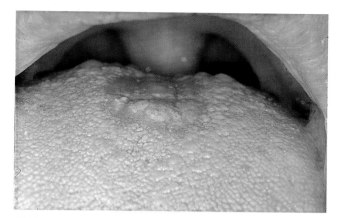

159. This patient felt he had contracted a 'disease' from a new sexual partner.

a. What is the diagnosis?
b. What is the management of this condition?

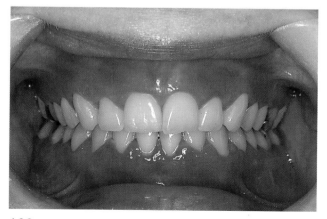

160. The patient shown here was concerned about painful, swollen gums despite vigorous oral hygiene.

a. What is the clinical description applied to this condition?
b. What advice would you give to this patient while pursuing a definitive diagnosis?

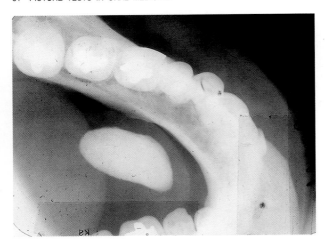

161. This patient reported swelling of the submandibular region around mealtimes, with a foul-tasting discharge in the mouth.

a. What has caused the swelling?
b. How should the patient be managed in the acute phase of this problem?
c. What longer-term treatment options are possible?

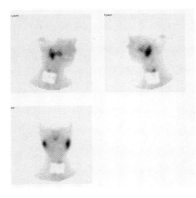

162. This special test may be used in the investigation of patients with putative dry mouth.

a. Name the special test.
b. What systemic diseases may be part of Sjögren's syndrome?
c. What serological markers may be evident in Sjögren's syndrome?

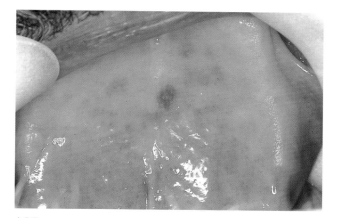

163. This area of pigmentation occurred in a businessman during a prolonged period overseas.

a. What drug is most likely to have caused this?
b. What other drugs may cause oral pigmentation?

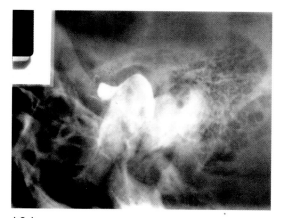

164. This radiographic film was obtained from a patient with symptoms of temporomandibular joint (TMJ) pain.

a. What condition is evident?
b. What important questions put to the patient might alert the clinician to such a problem, as distinct from classical TMJ dysfunction syndrome?

165. **This magnetic resonance imaging (MRI) scan was performed on a patient with trigeminal neuralgia.**

a. What intracerebral pathology was being excluded?
b. Describe the classical features of the pain associated with trigeminal neuralgia.
c. What drugs are available for the treatment of trigeminal neuralgia?

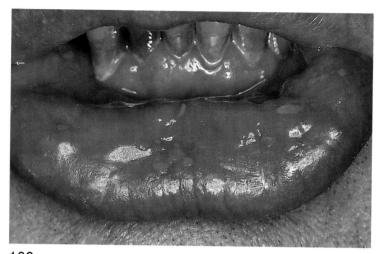

166. This patient presented with frequent attacks of painful 'pinhead' ulcers throughout the oral mucosa. These have occurred regularly for 20 years.

a. What is the diagnosis?
b. What particular treatment may be beneficial?

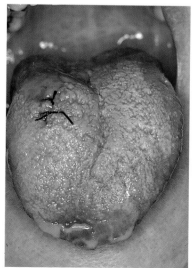

167. A 58-year-old female patient presented with painful 'blisters' in her mouth. Examination revealed erosive lesions and intact bullae with clear fluid inside.

a. What is the differential diagnosis?
b. What special tests would help you in making a definitive diagnosis?

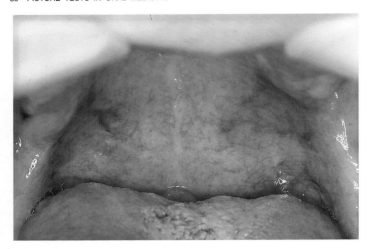

168. This patient has a history of poorly controlled hypertension and was recently started on appropriate drug therapy. These oral lesions appeared 10 days later.

a. What is the likely diagnosis?
b. What special investigations are warranted?
c. How should the patient be managed?

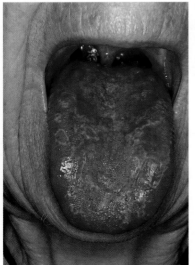

169. This lesion was described histologically as a 'lichenoid tissue eruption'.

a. What are the drug groups most likely to cause such a reaction?

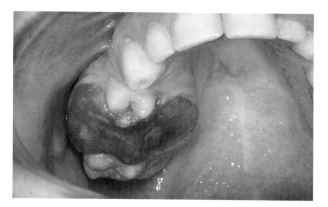

170. This appearance was noted in an HIV-positive patient some days after extraction of a loose upper molar tooth.

a. What diagnoses should be considered?
b. What investigations are appropriate?

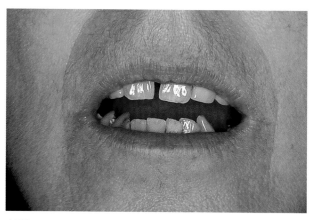

171. These chronic lip lesions have prompted this patient to seek help and advice.

a. What is the diagnosis?
b. What organisms are likely to be involved?
c. What microbiological samples are appropriate?

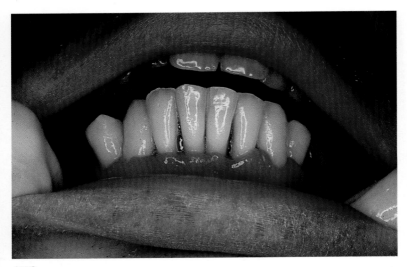

172. This gingival appearance was noted in an HIV-positive male patient.

a. What is the diagnosis?
b. Which areas of the mouth are most commonly affected?

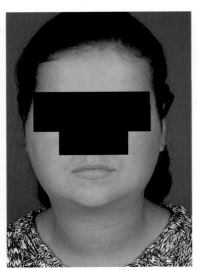

173. This female patient presented with a 48 hour history of increasing facial swelling bilaterally and profound pain. She was febrile and lethargic.

a. What is the likely diagnosis?
b. How should the patient be managed?

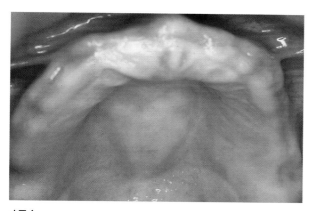

174. This palatal lump was noticed by the patient's new dentist, but the patient states that this has been present for years.

a. What is the diagnosis?
b. What treatment is required?

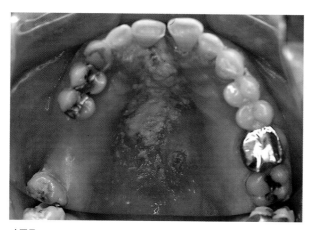

175. This middle-aged patient is in end-stage renal failure and this lesion was noted when he presented with an epistaxis.

a. What is the likely diagnosis?
b. What is the preferred therapy?

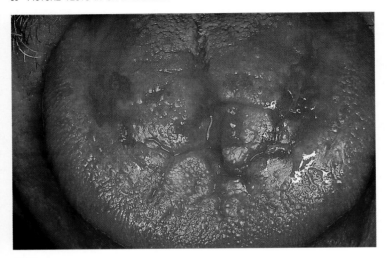

176. **This patient has troublesome ulcerated oral mucosal disease, diagnosed as lichen planus. Topical corticosteroid therapy has proved ineffective.**

a. What systemic agents are available to treat this condition?
b. List the potential side-effects of systemic corticosteroid therapy.

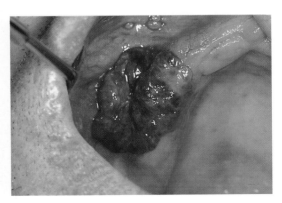

177. **This patient had a skin neoplasm removed some years previously.**

a. What is the likely diagnosis?
b. What is the likely prognosis?

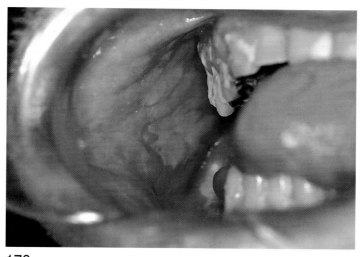

178. This 55-year-old male has recently undergone treatment for an oral carcinoma.

a. What clinical features are evident?
b. What is the diagnosis?
c. What treatment options are available?

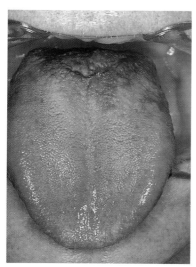

179. Following multiple medication for recurrent respiratory tract infections, this patient was referred for investigation of his asymptomatic tongue condition.

a. What is the diagnosis?
b. Is his past medical history pertinent?

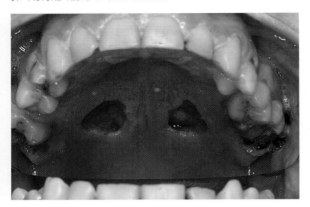

180. This 40-year-old patient, who smokes in excess of 40 cigarettes per day, presented with painless palatal lesions of 14 days duration.

a. What is the diagnosis?
b. What are considered to be the aetiological factors?
c. What other diagnosis might an inexperienced pathologist suggest on histological findings?

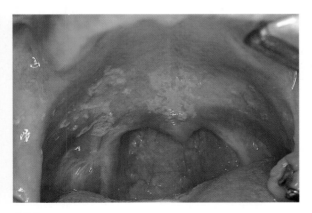

181. This patient has presented with florid intra-oral candidosis. He has expressed fears of HIV-related disease.

a. How would you manage this immediate situation?
b. What appropriate steps should be considered with respect to ongoing dental care?

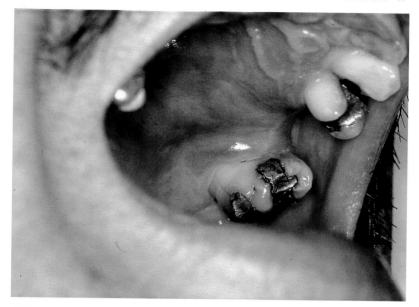

182. This patient is HIV-positive and has developed a lesion on his palate.

a. What is the diagnosis?
b. What is known about the aetiology of this lesion?

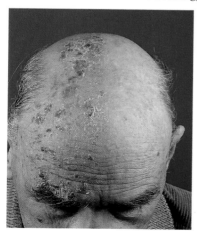

183. This 60-year-old man subsequently developed severe pain in the right side of his forehead which was not controlled by potent analgesic drugs.

a. What is the diagnosis?
b. How might he be managed?

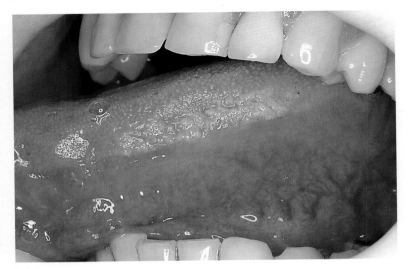

184. **This HIV-positive patient has a lesion affecting the side of his tongue.**

a. What is the diagnosis?
b. What management is appropriate?

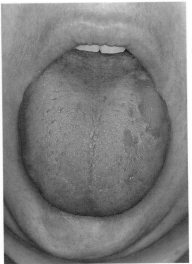

185. **This patient who is attending with a geographic tongue has developed a dry mouth since changing her antihypertensive medication.**

a. What drugs can cause dryness of the oral mucosa?
b. How may this situation be managed?

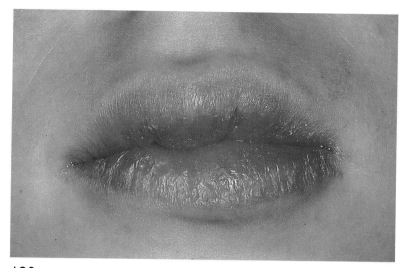

186. This patient developed swelling of the lips and angular cheilitis.

a. How may dietary factors influence this clinical presentation?

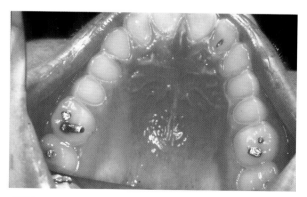

187. This 28-year-old female patient is under psychiatric care for an eating disorder.

a. What clinical features are evident?
b. What is the likely diagnosis?
c. What dental treatment options are possible?

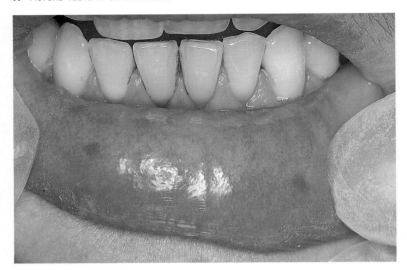

188. This patient developed widespread intra-oral melanosis over a few weeks. She felt generally unwell with weight loss and dizziness.

a. What important systemic disease should be excluded?
b. What physical test performed at the chairside would be helpful in diagnosis?
c. What blood tests would be helpful in diagnosis?

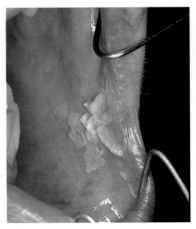

189. This 60-year-old male patient experienced some discomfort at his labial commissures after his dentist had attempted to take impressions.

a. What is the diagnosis?
b. What is the significance of this lesion?

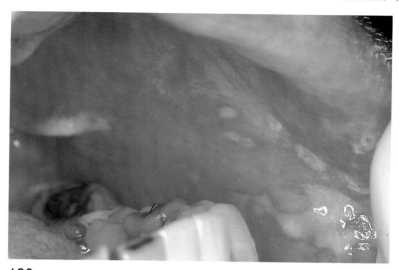

190. This patient had associated skin lesions affecting the mandibular division of the left trigeminal nerve.

a. What is the likely diagnosis?
b. What determines the distribution of the lesions?

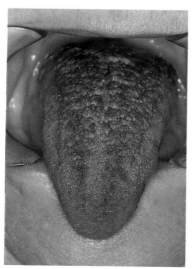

191. This tongue condition was observed in a 60-year-old male patient with a history of alcohol and tobacco misuse.

a. What is the diagnosis?
b. How may his social habits have contributed to this appearance?

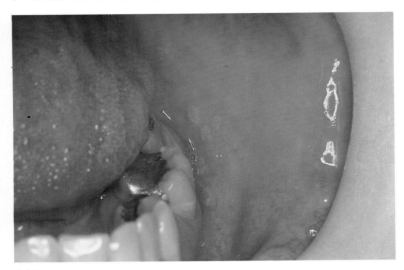

192. These yellow-coloured spots were noticed by a patient who was deeply concerned about sinister pathology in her mouth.

a. What is the diagnosis?
b. How common are these?

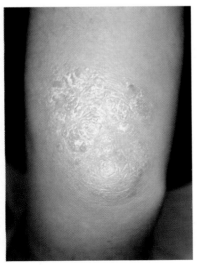

193. This patient has a common skin condition.

a. What is the diagnosis?
b. What do the oral lesions in this condition resemble?

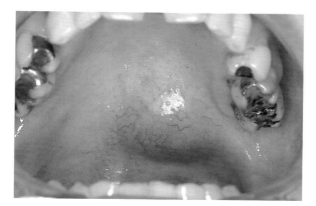

194. This palatal swelling, present for 3 months, was painless. Biopsy revealed it to be a salivary gland tumour.

a. What are the most common benign salivary gland tumours?
b. What is the most common malignant salivary gland tumour and how does it spread?

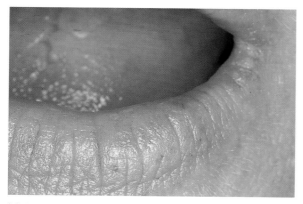

195. This patient's lip lesions have failed to resolve with antibiotics prescribed by her general medical practitioner.

a. What associated intra-oral pathology might you expect to see, given that this patient is a wearer of complete dentures?
b. What investigations are appropriate for this patient?
c. What topical treatments are available?

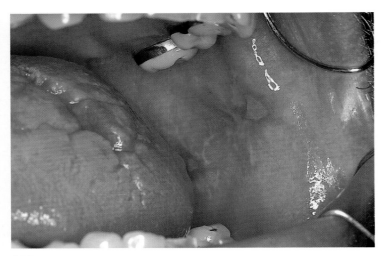

196. This patient, a regular attender at the dentist, developed this lesion adjacent to a large, aged amalgam restoration.

a. What is the clinical diagnosis?
b. What investigations are appropriate if the patient's lesions are symptomatic?

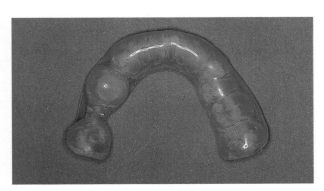

197. This appliance is used in the management of myofascial pain dysfunction syndrome (MPDS).

a. What is the appliance?
b. Describe the classical symptoms in MPDS.
c. What other treatment options may be considered?

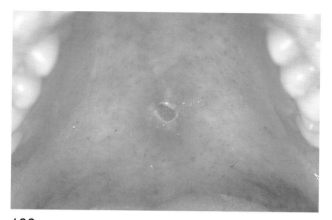

198. The clinical photograph shows evidence of ulceration of the hard palate in a female patient with muscle and joint pain and photosensitive skin eruptions.

a. What is the likely diagnosis?
b. How may the oral lesions be managed?

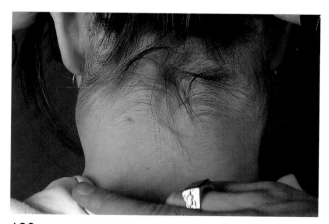

199. This 17-year-old woman presented with bilateral painless neck swellings of 4 weeks duration.

a. What is the differential diagnosis?
b. How should this patient be managed?

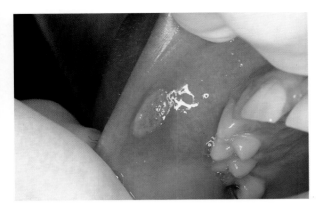

200. **This female patient has developed cyclical recurrent aphthous stomatitis.**

a. During which phase of the menstrual cycle are aphthae most likely to occur?

b. What effect is pregnancy likely to have on these ulcers?

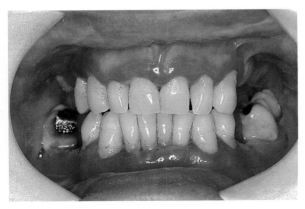

201. **This patient has discomfort and bleeding from her gingivae despite impeccable oral hygiene.**

a. What descriptive term is used for this type of lesion?

b. The histology suggests subepithelial splitting. What further investigations are indicated?

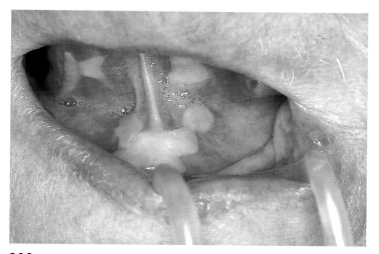

202. This patient has a blistering condition which affects the mouth and genitalia.

a. What group of disorders does the condition belong to?
b. What investigations should be carried out?
c. What other body sites should be examined by the appropriate specialist?

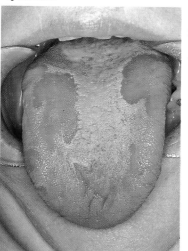

203. This tongue lesion was persistent but entirely painless.

a. What is the diagnosis?
b. How should the patient be managed?

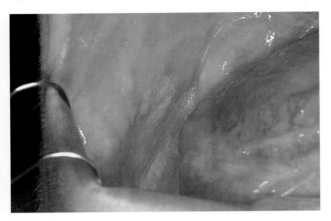

204. A 40-year-old female patient presents with a long-standing white patch of the buccal mucosa. Biopsy suggests moderate to severe epithelial dysplasia.

a. How should the patient be managed?
b. What long-term plans should be instituted for this patient?

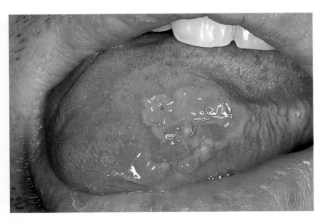

205. This HIV-positive patient has a persistent, painful ulcer on the left side of his tongue.

a. What is the likely diagnosis?
b. What treatment is available?

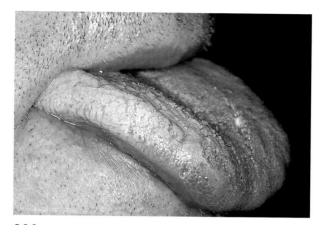

206. This patient was using aspirin to alleviate toothache.

a. What is the diagnosis?
b. How should the patient be managed?

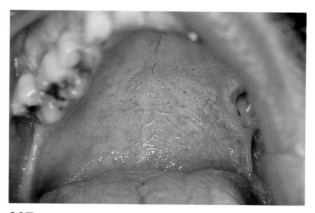

207. This appearance on the palate of a 50-year-old male was noticed at routine dental examination. He smokes pipe tobacco.

a. What is the diagnosis?
b. What is the nature of the red spots?

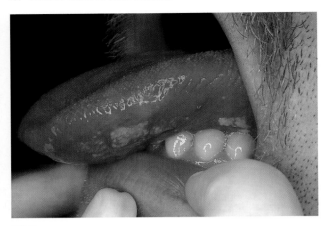

208. **This tongue lesion appeared relatively quickly in an HIV-positive patient.**

a. What is the likely diagnosis?
b. What other diagnoses should be considered?

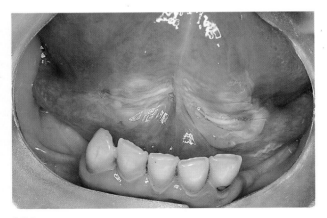

209. **This lesion was noted in a life-long smoker.**

a. What is the diagnosis?
b. What management should be instituted for this patient?
c. Why is the clinical site important?

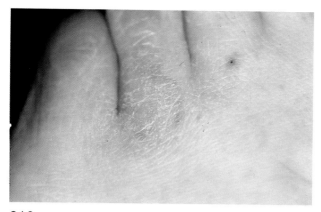

210. A patient with chronic oral candidosis used his prescribed medication in an attempt to treat his foot lesion.

a. What is the likely diagnosis?
b. Is there any link with his oral condition?
c. Why was the medication unhelpful in treating his foot?

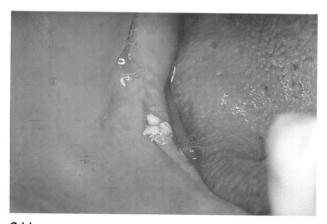

211. There were several of these exophytic lesions in the mouth of an HIV-positive male patient.

a. What is the diagnosis?
b. What is the causative agent?
c. How may this be demonstrated?

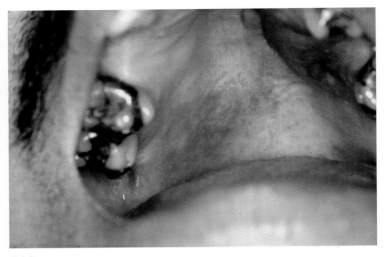

212. This palatal lesion was noticed by an HIV-positive patient who diagnosed the condition himself.

a. What is the diagnosis?
b. Is this a common site for this condition?

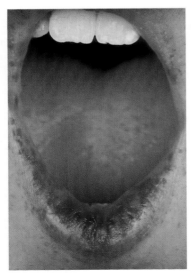

213. This young boy has an associated gastrointestinal abnormality.

a. What is the diagnosis?
b. What lesions are found in the gastrointestinal tract, and where?
c. What is the inheritance pattern of this condition?

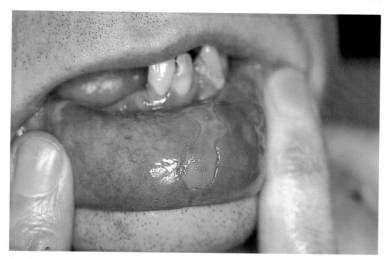

214. This ulceration was noted in a patient with active Crohn's disease.

a. What is the diagnosis?
b. What other types of oral ulceration might be seen in patients with inflammatory bowel disease?

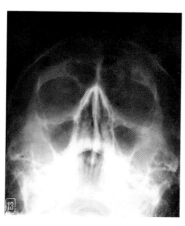

215. This radiograph was taken to exclude antral pathology in a 28-year-old female patient with a 1 year history of a constant dull ache affecting the upper right quadrant.

a. What is the diagnosis?
b. How should the patient be managed?

Answers

1. a. Denture stomatitis (chronic erythematous candidosis).
   b. Microbiological culture can demonstrate the presence of *Candida* spp. but not the presence of active infection.
   c. The diagnosis is confirmed by a positive response to antifungal therapy and denture hygiene instruction.

2. a. The forehead is supplied by both ipsilateral and contralateral nerve fibres, and hence the lack of wrinkling of the forehead implies that this is a lower motor neurone lesion.
   b. This is most likely to be a Bell's palsy.
   c. Systemic corticosteroids are only effective if given within 72 hours of the onset of the palsy, so the appropriate treatment at 2 weeks is conservative.

3. a. She is likely also to complain of a dry mouth.
   b. Secondary Sjögren's syndrome is seen in association with a connective tissue disorder, most commonly rheumatoid arthritis.

4. a. Erythema multiforme.
   b. The bullae are largely subepithelial.
   c. The condition is an immune complex disorder and may be precipitated by a herpes simplex infection or by drugs.

5. a. Herpetic gingivostomatitis.
   b. This diagnosis may be confirmed by demonstrating virus from a swab or smear by immunofluorescence or by showing a fourfold rise in anti-herpes-simplex antibodies in the convalescent serum.

6. a. Minor recurrent aphthous stomatitis.
   b. The hard palate and attached gingivae are not affected by aphthae.
   c. The female:male ratio is approximately 1.5 : 1.

7. a. Orofacial granulomatosis.
   b. This may be an oral manifestation of Crohn's disease or sarcoidosis.

8. a. Clinically this is most likely to be a squamous cell carcinoma.
   b. Biopsy is confirmatory.
   c. Smoking and alcohol consumption in combination greatly increase the risk of developing oral malignancy.
   d. The carcinoma can be treated by surgery or radiotherapy either alone or in combination.

9. a. Trauma or syphilitic chancre.
   b. Syphilis serology and biopsy of the lesion.

10. a. Clinically, this is an haemangioma. It has increased in size clinically over the last 2 years not because of an increase in the absolute size of the lesion, but because it has become more superficial.
    b. If the lesion is troublesome, it can be surgically excised or treated with cryotherapy or laser surgery.
    c. If this lesion is traumatised, it may bleed profusely.

11. a. This condition is angina bullosa haemorrhagica.
    b. Immunofluorescence is negative in this condition.
    c. Because of the self-limiting nature of this condition, reassurance is all that is required. Patients should, however, avoid traumatising their palate with rough food if possible.

12. a. This is an epulis associated with pregnancy gingivitis.
    b. The immediate management is to scale and polish the region and reinforce oral hygiene instruction. Excision alone will lead to recurrence unless the underlying stimulus is removed.
    c. The condition is likely to resolve spontaneously post-partum.

13. a. Clinically, this is likely to be a hairy leukoplakia.
    b. Histologically, this will show an irregular hyperkeratotic epithelium, usually with candidal infestation and koilocyte-like cells in the epithelium. There will be no associated submucosal inflammatory response.
    c. The diagnosis of hairy leukoplakia can be confirmed by the demonstration of Epstein–Barr virus within the epithelium using in situ hybridisation.

14. a. Clinically, this is reticular lichen planus.
    b. A biopsy is required to confirm the diagnosis.
    c. Since this condition is asymptomatic, the patient requires only reassurance and review.

15. a. This patient has tori mandibularis.
    b. These lesions are likely to increase slowly over time.
    c. Unless they become mechanically obtrusive, these lesions should be left.

16. a. This patient shows palatal erosion of her upper anterior teeth.
    b. The distribution suggests that this is erosion from stomach acid entering the mouth during recurrent vomiting, and it is therefore most likely to be due to bulimia nervosa.
    c. The patient should be referred via her general medical practitioner for specialist care of her bulimia and her dentition should be restored.

17.
a. This patient has glossitis.
b. It would be appropriate in the first instance to examine her haematologically. The appropriate tests would be a full blood count, serum ferritin, folate and vitamin B_{12} levels.
c. A patient who is nutritionally deficient with glossitis may also be susceptible to aphthae and angular cheilitis.

18.
a. This patient is suffering from smoker's palate.
b. This is due to irritation of the palate from either cigarette or pipe tobacco smoke.
c. Although the lesion has a low risk of malignant transformation, the patient should be encouraged to stop smoking.

19.
a. This patient probably has a traumatic ulcer.
b. Any obvious cause for the trauma should be removed and the patient should be reassured, given symptomatic therapy and reviewed.

20.
a. This patient has an amalgam tattoo.
b. The amalgam may be visible radiographically or it can be visualised on histological examination.
c. The patient requires reassurance only.

21.
a. This photograph is of a parotid sialogram.
b. The sialogram shows features of sialectasis or a 'snowstorm' appearance.
c. Patients who have an acute salivary gland infection should not have a sialogram performed until the infection is brought under control. Iodine hypersensitivity is also a contraindication.

22.
a. This patient has a mucocutaneous bullous disorder which may be pemphigoid or pemphigus.
b. A tissue sample and venous blood are required for direct and indirect immunofluorescence, respectively.
c. In the case of pemphigoid, immunofluorescence would be along the basement membrane zone, whereas in pemphigus the immunofluorescence would be suprabasal.

23.
a. This patient is suffering from angular cheilitis.
b. Angular cheilitis may arise from a combination of infection associated with a reduced vertical dimension, skin folding or systemic disease such as diabetes mellitus or nutritional deficiencies. The patient is also likely to have chronic erythematous candidosis.

24.
a. This white patch on the floor of the patient's mouth may be initiated and exacerbated in some cases by alcohol and tobacco use.

b. Biopsy for histological examination is essential in this case.

25.
a. Systemic lupus erythematosus.
b. Histological features include para- or orthokeratosis, liquefaction degeneration of the basal cell layer, hyalinisation of the subepithelial connective tissue, and a chronic inflammatory cell infiltrate in the subepithelial connective tissue, often with a perivascular distribution. An overt vasculitis may be evident.

26.
a. Lichen planus will show epithelial atrophy with or without hyperkeratosis or ulceration, Civatte bodies, liquefactive degeneration, loss of rete ridges and a hugging band of lymphocytes in the submucosa.
b. Lichen planus affecting the dorsal or lateral borders of the tongue or the gingivae is more likely to become malignant (1–2%) than lichen planus in other parts of the mouth. Similarly, erosive and atrophic variants have a higher risk of malignant transformation.

27.
a. This patient has an intra-oral herpes zoster infection.
b. If the patient is seen within the first 72 hours of the clinical appearance of this infection, it is appropriate to give aciclovir 800 mg five times daily for 7 days, and this may shorten the clinical course of the infection and prevent post-herpetic neuralgia. The patient should also be given suitable analgesia.

28.
a. Clinically, this patient has a candidal leukoplakia.
b. This must be confirmed by biopsy.
c. Patients with candidal leukoplakia are inevitably smokers.

29.
a. Clinically, this patient is most likely to have a pleomorphic salivary adenoma affecting the parotid gland.
b. This could be confirmed histologically using fine-needle aspiration. If this failed, open biopsy would be required.
c. The appropriate treatment for such a lesion, if confirmed to be a pleomorphic salivary adenoma, would be a superficial parotidectomy, since the majority of pleomorphic salivary adenomas affect the superficial part of the gland. Enucleation would be unsatisfactory.

30.
a. This patient suffers from minor recurrent aphthous stomatitis.
b. Initially the patient should be investigated haematologically by having a full blood count and assays of serum ferritin, folate and serum vitamin B_{12} levels carried out.
c. A deficiency of iron, folic acid or vitamin B_{12} occurs singly or in combination in 20% of patients presenting with recurrent aphthous stomatitis. Replacement therapy is usually attended by an improvement in, or remission of the ulceration.

31.
a. This is most likely to be a fibroepithelial polyp.
b. This lesion is not premalignant.
c. Simple surgical excision is the appropriate treatment.

32.
a. This patient has geographic tongue (erythema migrans).
b. Psoriasis.
c. Erythema migrans occurs in other parts of the mouth in addition to the tongue.

33.
a. This patient has pseudomembranous candidosis.
b. In an apparently fit young man, HIV infection and diabetes mellitus should be considered as an underlying cause for this clinical appearance.
c. A potassium hydroxide or Gram's stain smear of one of the white plaques would demonstrate epithelial squames and fungal mycelia.

34.
a. Pemphigus vulgaris is an organ-specific autoimmune disease with antibodies directed against the intercellular cementing substance of the prickle cell layer.
b. The immunofluorescent features show basket-weave staining suprabasally, usually with IgM, IgG and C3.
c. Treatment consists of systemic corticosteroids with or without steroid-sparing agents such as azathioprine.

35.
a. This pigmented lesion requires biopsy for diagnosis. In this case, a melanotic macule was diagnosed.
b. The brown coloration is melanin present both in the melanocytes and in melanosomes contained in submucosal macrophages.

36.
a. A full blood count should be carried out on this patient to exclude leukaemia.
b. Leukaemia would also be associated with pallor due to anaemia, bruising due to thrombocytopenia, generalised lymphadenopathy and hepatosplenomegaly.

37.
a. This lesion is most likely to be a salivary gland neoplasm, since mucoceles are uncommon in the upper lip.
b. Excision biopsy is indicated.

38.
a. This is likely to be a white sponge naevus.
b. This could be confirmed by biopsy.
c. The patient requires only reassurance.

39.
a. This is direct immunofluorescence since it shows in vivo bound antibodies in a biopsy from a patient.
b. This patient has pemphigus, because the immunofluorescence is directed against the intercellular cementing substance of the prickle cell layer.

c. Although the condition may present exclusively as an oral problem, because she has pemphigus this patient is likely to develop skin lesions as well.

40.
a. This is median rhomboid glossitis.
b. Asthmatic patients who inhale corticosteroids are predisposed to median rhomboid glossitis, due to local immunosuppression.
c. Median rhomboid glossitis represents a form of erythematous candidosis and therefore *Candida albicans* is the most likely causative agent.

41.
a. This patient may have Peutz–Jeghers syndrome and may therefore have intestinal polyposis.
b. A barium meal and follow-through would visualise the polyposis, but endoscopy would be required for histological diagnosis.
c. There is a small likelihood of intestinal obstruction but there is a low malignant transformation rate in Peutz–Jeghers syndrome.

42.
a. This patient has a black hairy tongue.
b. The condition often arises apparently spontaneously but may arise subsequent to antibiotic therapy.
c. The condition is treated mechanically by brushing the tongue with a toothbrush and with the use of a peroxide or perborate mouthwash.

43.
a. This patient has a herpes labialis lesion or a 'cold sore'.
b. This is caused by a herpes simplex virus.
c. This patient should be informed that the lesion is infectious. The patient may use a desiccating agent such as alcohol to encourage eschar formation. In the prodromal phase, the lesion can be treated with aciclovir 5% cream five times daily.

44.
a. This patient may have developed intra-oral pigmentation secondary to a drug reaction, e.g. antimalarials, or may be developing Addison's disease.
b. A normal Synacthen test, which measures the patient's adrenal response to adrenocorticotrophic hormone, would exclude the diagnosis of Addison's disease.

45.
a. The most useful investigations for excluding sarcoidosis are a chest radiograph to exclude hilar lymphadenopathy and measurement of the serum angiotensin-converting enzyme level, which may be elevated in sarcoidosis.
b. A barium radiograph would be useful in excluding associated gut Crohn's disease.

46.
a. This is likely to be cutaneous lichen planus.
b. The phenomenon of developing a lesion secondary to trauma or irritation is called the Koebner phenomenon.
c. Thirty per cent of patients with skin lichen planus also have oral lichen planus.

47.
a. Fissured or scrotal tongue.
b. This entity is most often seen in patients with no obvious causation. It is also associated with Down syndrome, geographic tongue and the Melkersson–Rosenthal syndrome.
c. Management includes reassurance, topical anaesthetic agents or benzydamine hydrochloride rinse. The fissures should be swabbed for possible microbiological growth, especially *Candida* spp.

48.
a. This patient has a clinical diagnosis of sialosis.
b. This may be associated with diabetes mellitus, protein malnutrition or alcoholism. It is most commonly idiopathic.
c. The sialographic appearances are normal.

49.
a. This patient has frictional keratoses due to cheek chewing.
b. This is not likely to show any features of epithelial dysplasia.
c. Frictional or smoking keratoses are usually associated with a minimal inflammatory cell infiltrate.

50.
a. Newton classified denture stomatitis as follows: I, pinpoint erythema which may be traumatic in nature; II, diffuse erythema of the denture-bearing area; III, papilliferous overgrowth of the mucosa covering the palate under the fitting surface of the denture.
b. Chronic erythematous candidosis is amenable to topical treatment with amphotericin, nystatin or miconazole.

51.
a. This is a squamous cell carcinoma.
b. This lesion is likely to spread locally and then to the regional lymph nodes.

52.
a. This patient suffers from rheumatoid arthritis.
b. The patient's hand shows swelling of the metacarpophalangeal joints, atrophy of the small muscles of the hand, and a buttonhole deformity of the interphalangeal joints.

53.
a. This patient has Fordyce spots.
b. These are ectopic sebaceous glands.
c. Reassurance is all that is required.

54.
a. This patient has denture stomatitis or chronic erythematous candidosis.
b. The denture acts as a reservoir for the infecting agent.

Furthermore, ill-fitting dentures may traumatise the mucosa and aggravate the clinical condition.

  c. The vast majority of patients can have *Candida* spp. isolated from the lesion, although occasionally a bacterial or mixed infection may present in this way.

55.
  a. The most common causes of a dry mouth are drugs, particularly tricylic antidepressants, chronic anxiety and Sjögren's syndrome.

  b. Patients with xerostomia are susceptible to caries, gingivitis and candidosis.

56.
  a. This patient has erythema multiforme.

  b. If the diagnosis is in doubt, biopsy is usually confirmatory.

  c. The condition may be self-limiting but often requires systemic corticosteroids. Some patients develop erythema multiforme as a reaction to a herpes infection and prophylactic aciclovir may be beneficial.

57.
  a. This patient has primary herpetic gingivostomatitis.

  b. This can be distinguished from recurrent aphthae as recurrent oral ulcers do not affect the attached gingivae.

  c. If the patient presents within 2 days of onset, aciclovir 200 mg five times daily for 5 days may shorten the course of the infection.

58.
  a. There is evidence of a genetic component to recurrent oral ulceration: first-degree relatives of patients with aphthae are far more likely also to be sufferers and there is a mild HLA association (A2 and B12).

  b. Patients who smoke are relatively protected from recurrent oral ulceration and they often develop recurrent oral ulcers for the first time on giving up cigarette smoking.

59.
  a. This patient suffers from Melkersson–Rosenthal syndrome.

  b. It is thought that the facial nerve palsy arises as a result of pressure on the nerve from granuloma formation.

60.
  a. Cigarette smoking and alcohol consumption each compound the other's effects as a carcinogen.

  b. You should explain to the patient that she will be seen at a joint clinic with a radiotherapist and surgeon to determine the best therapeutic approach.

  c. You should examine this patient clinically for evidence of regional lymphadenopathy, which would imply metastatic spread of the carcinoma. In addition, specialist radiological scanning is indicated.

61.
  a. A coagulation screen and full blood count should be carried out in consultation with the local haematology department.

b. If the patient is on warfarin, his/her INR (international normalised ratio) should be reduced below 2.5 before an extraction is carried out.

62.
a. Clinically, this patient has a lingual tonsillitis.
b. The patient should be examined for other tonsillar or nodal involvement.
c. The patient is likely to recover with symptomatic therapy alone, without the need for antibiotics.

63.
a. This patient has a bullous disorder which is most likely to be pemphigoid.
b. Immunofluorescence in this patient will show deposition of IgM, IgG and/or C3 along the basement membrane zone.
c. The patient is likely to need systemic corticosteroids in the first instance to bring the disease under control, but may then be controlled with topical corticosteroids.

64.
a. This patient has fibrous hyperplasia of the gingivae, which is most often due to phenytoin, cyclosporin or calcium channel blockers.
b. Scrupulous oral hygiene usually improves the situation but gingivectomy may be required to reduce unsightly overgrowth. Cessation of drug therapy is not usually an option.

65.
a. This patient has a sublingual keratosis.
b. The patient should be asked about smoking and drinking habits.
c. This patient requires a biopsy to assess the presence and degree of epithelial dysplasia.

66.
a. This patient has erosive lichen planus or lichenoid eruption.
b. This may be a lichenoid reaction to drugs, foodstuffs or amalgam.
c. Identification of the cause is the first line of investigation. The mainstay of treatment is topical corticosteroid therapy.

67.
a. This patient has common warts on his finger and lip.
b. Human papilloma virus.
c. Surgical excision or cryotherapy.

68.
a. This patient has gross caries secondary to radiation-induced xerostomia.
b. Deterioration can be halted by improving oral hygiene and by the use of topical applications of fluoride. Fluoride-containing saliva substitutes may also be of benefit.
c. This patient then requires advanced restorative treatment to maintain the dentition. Wearing removable prostheses may be problematic.

69.
 a. This patient does not require any active therapy since she is asymptomatic.
 b. Longitudinal ridging of the nails may occur in lichen planus.

70.
 a. This man has an atrophic glossitis and may have an associated dysphagia due to an oesophageal web, since glossitis and dysphagia can occur concurrently in Brown–Kelly–Patterson syndrome.
 b. This is associated with iron deficiency anaemia.
 c. There is an increased risk of oesophageal carcinoma in these patients.

71.
 a. The most likely diagnosis in this patient's case is a melanotic macule, although a more sinister lesion cannot be ruled out clinically.
 b. It is therefore necessary to biopsy this patient to exclude malignant melanoma.

72.
 a. The sialogram shows a stricture of the parotid duct.
 b. This patient should be treated with dilation of the parotid duct. The patient should also be encouraged to flush the salivary glands out each morning using an acidic drink and massaging the gland.

73.
 a. Osteogenesis imperfecta, which is associated with blue sclerae.
 b. Dentinogenesis imperfecta.

74.
 a. This patient has angular cheilitis.
 b. In a dentate young boy, the most likely infective agents are *Staphylococcus* or *Streptococcus*.
 c. In the first instance, empirical therapy with miconazole cream should be used.

75.
 a. This patient has desquamative gingivitis.
 b. Desquamative gingivitis may be caused by lichen planus, bullous disorders, plasma cell (allergic) gingivitis or psoriasis.
 c. Biopsy of non-marginal gingivae is required to establish the diagnosis. Thereafter, corticosteroids are the mainstay of therapy, used either as a spray or mouthwash or under an occlusive veneer or splint.

76.
 a. Clinically, this patient has lupus erythematosus, which characteristically affects the palate.
 b. This diagnosis can be confirmed by biopsy.
 c. A blood test for antinuclear factor as part of an autoantibody screen would be helpful.

77.
 a. Clinically, this patient has a candidal leukoplakia.
 b. Histological confirmation is required, which will also indicate the degree of epithelial dysplasia.

    c. Treatment comprises persuading the patient to give up smoking and providing him with a systemic antifungal agent such as fluconazole 50 mg daily for 2 weeks.

78.
a. This patient has a trigeminal herpes zoster infection.
b. This could be confirmed by direct culture of vesicular fluid or by immunofluorescence of vesicular fluid.
c. This patient's pain is likely to resolve when the lesions resolve or within a few weeks thereafter.

79.
a. This patient has a major aphthous ulcer.
b. If clinical doubt persists, a biopsy would be warranted.
c. Pain relief with a topical anaesthetic spray is indicated and the patient should use an antiseptic mouthwash, such as chlorhexidine, and a topical corticosteroid.

80.
a. This patient has median rhomboid glossitis.
b. This could be confirmed histologically although the clinical diagnosis should suffice.
c. Smoking and the use of corticosteroid aerosol sprays may precipitate the condition, as may diabetes mellitus or HIV infection.
d. No treatment is required if the patient is asymptomatic. Clinical and symptomatic improvement will occur with systemic antifungal agents such as fluconazole.

81.
a. This child should use a prophylactic 0.2% chlorhexidine mouthwash twice daily. He should also use topical antifungal agents.
b. A painful, carious premolar in this child should be excavated and dressed with a sedative dressing, and definitive treatment should be deferred until after induction of a remission, if symptoms permit.

82.
a. This is a mucocele.
b. This lesion should be excised along with the underlying damaged minor salivary gland.
c. Histologically it will show an epithelial-lined cyst if it is a mucous retention cyst, or it will show a macrophage-lined cavity filled with saliva if it is a mucous extravasation cyst.

83.
a. This is most likely to have been caused by a piece of amalgam in a healed extraction socket, the so-called 'amalgam tattoo'.
b. If amalgam tattoo is suspected, a simple radiograph will reveal the offending object. However, biopsy is essential for all other areas of oral pigmentation and if the radiograph reveals nothing.

84.
a. The diagnosis is geographic tongue, also known as erythema migrans and benign migratory glossitis.

    b. It is largely idiopathic but is also said to be associated with psoriasis and Reiter's syndrome.

    c. Management includes reassurance, topical anaesthetic agents or benzydamine hydrochloride rinse. There is some evidence that it may be associated with zinc deficiency in some patients and so this should be excluded by a blood test. Appropriate zinc replacement therapy may result in resolution of the clinical appearance and symptoms.

85.
    a. Clinically, this is a frictional keratosis.

    b. This patient should have a biopsy performed and reviewed periodically.

86.
    a. This lesion occurs as a result of reactivation of latent herpes simplex viral infection in the trigeminal ganglion.

    b. Reactivation may be caused by trauma, UV light, cyclical hormone changes, stress or systemic illness.

87.
    a. The oral manifestations of orofacial granulomatosis are lip swelling (with or without fissuring), cobblestoning of the buccal mucosa, localised tissue swellings, full-thickness gingivitis, mucosal tags, linear ulcers, angular cheilitis and recurrent aphthae.

88.
    a. Clinically, this patient has lichen planus.

    b. The patient may have cutaneous lichen planus, although lichen planus has not been consistently shown to be associated with any other systemic disorder.

89.
    a. This patient has an eruption cyst.

    b. The roof can be taken off the cyst surgically.

    c. Histologically, the excised portion would show an epithelial-lined cavity which had arisen from the reduced enamel epithelium.

90.
    a. This patient has a candidal leukoplakia.

    b. The histological section should be stained with Periodic Acid Schiff to highlight the candidal hyphae.

91.
    a. It is important to exclude leukaemia as a diagnosis in this patient.

    b. This can be done simply by examining a full blood count.

    c. The patient is likely to be susceptible to intra-oral infection (viral and fungal), gingival swelling, spontaneous haemorrhage, and occasionally swellings due to leukaemic deposits. Patients may also develop leukaemic ulceration.

92.
    a. These are target lesions.

    b. This is most likely to be erythema multiforme.

93.
a. Clinically, this is lupus erythematosus.
b. This condition may be subdivided into systemic or discoid lupus erythematosus.
c. If the lesion is symptomatic, treatment with topical corticosteroids is warranted.

94.
a. This patient has acute necrotising ulcerative gingivitis.
b. This presents as painful, bleeding gums which clinically reveal a characteristic fetor oris, necrosis of the tips of the interdental papillae and cratering interproximally.
c. This is a co-infection with spirochaetes and fusiform bacilli.
d. Necrotising ulcerative gingivitis may be a manifestation of HIV infection.

95.
a. This boy is likely to have cyclic neutropenia.
b. Repeated daily white cell counts, over a period of 2–3 weeks, are necessary to make the diagnosis.
c. The condition is idiopathic but involves an abnormality of neutrophil production.

96.
a. Clinically, this patient has a smoker's palate.
b. The oral cavity should be carefully examined to exclude premalignant or malignant lesions, related to smoking.

97.
a. The photograph shows a ranula.
b. The most common cause of a ranula is a blocked sublingual gland.
c. Treatment involves laying open the roof of the ranula or collapsing it by aspirating the saliva contents.

98.
a. This patient has a torus palatinus.
b. This may be associated with mandibular tori.

99.
a. This patient has cutaneous lichen planus.
b. Twenty per cent of patients with oral lesions have skin lesions as well.
c. Skin lesions tend to resolve within 18 months.

100.
a. She is likely to have vitamin B_{12} deficiency since Crohn's disease affects the terminal ileum ('regional ileitis') where vitamin B_{12} is absorbed.
b. She should have her putative deficiency state investigated and corrected.

101.
a. Clinically, this young boy has herpangina.
b. This is due to a Coxsackie virus infection.
c. Coxsackie virus may also cause hand, foot and mouth disease.

102.
a. The causative virus has most probably been auto-inoculated from a hand wart.

b. Surgical excision is the treatment of choice.

103.
a. This patient has a herpes zoster infection.
b. This may be associated with post-herpetic neuralgia.

104.
a. This photograph shows intra-oral pigmentation and hyperplastic candidosis. The patient has candidal endocrinopathy syndrome.
b. The pigmented lesions are due to Addison's disease.
c. The white lesions can be improved by prescribing a systemic antifungal agent.

105.
a. This person has developed rampant caries as a result of xerostomia induced by radiation.
b. Loss of the protective effects of saliva has caused excessive demineralisation.

106.
a. This patient had Crohn's disease.
b. He has a glossitis associated with vitamin B_{12} deficiency.
c. This patient requires blood investigations to confirm his deficiency state. Life-long parenteral vitamin B_{12} replacement therapy may well be indicated.

107.
a. This patient has a recurrent herpes simplex lesion of the face.
b. It is more usual to have this lesion on the vermilion border.

108.
a. The picture shows a discharging sinus arising from a periapical abscess in a mandibular molar.
b. *Actinomyces* may be the infecting organism in this case.
c. If actinomycosis is confirmed by microbiological examination, then prolonged penicillin therapy is warranted.

109.
a. This patient has tetracycline staining of the teeth.
b. The incremental pattern suggests the patient had been given tetracycline from the ages of 5 to 8 years.
c. Anterior veneers could be used to improve the aesthetics.

110.
a. The diagnosis is Gardner's syndrome.
b. This is an autosomal dominant disorder.
c. It is associated with colonic polyposis.
d. There is a high risk of malignant transformation, and prophylactic colectomy is often warranted.

111.
a. Angioedema.
b. Immediate hypersensitivity to the dentist's latex gloves or to a dental material.
c. Systemic antihistamines and close observation.

112.
a. The possible diagnoses are ethnic, drugs (e.g. oral contraceptive), irritational (e.g. smoking), Addison's disease, pigmented naevus, melanoma, amalgam tattoo, HIV-related and idiopathic.

b. A detailed history should be obtained, with particular reference to drugs and smoking; a detailed examination of the skin, mucous membranes and body systems (including blood pressure) should be carried out. A biopsy is essential. This case was a simple smoker's melanosis.

113.
a. This demonstrates globular sialectasis, indicative of Sjögren's syndrome.
b. There may be dryness of the oral mucosa with frothy saliva. The mucosa is thin and friable. Oral candidosis or staphylococcal infections are often problematic. There may be lobulation and depapillation of the tongue dorsum and an increased level of caries.

114.
a. Erythema multiforme, showing classical target or iris lesions.
b. Several predisposing factors are suggested, including herpes simplex and *Mycoplasma pneumoniae* infections, various drugs (including carbamazepine, codeine, penicillins, sulphonamides, tetracyclines and the thiazide diuretics), pregnancy, irradiation and internal malignancy.

115.
a. A fibro-epithelial polyp—the so-called 'leaf fibroma'.
b. Chronic irritation from the upper denture. The 'leaf' appearance is due to compression of the polyp.
c. Excision and provision of a new denture.

116.
a. Chronic erythematous candidosis.
b. Appropriate investigations may include microbiological sampling, and a random blood glucose assay (or at least urinalysis for glucose) should be performed.
c. Non-drug measures would include denture hygiene advice, the soaking of dentures overnight in hypochlorite solution (if there are no metal components) or chlorhexidine solution, and a reduction in the carbohydrate component of the diet. Ill-fitting dentures should be replaced.

117.
a. This appearance is highly consistent with a lichenoid drug eruption.
b. This is most likely due to ingested medication, particularly non-steroidal anti-inflammatories or antihypertensives.
c. Consultation with the patient's physician may allow alteration of the drug therapy, or alternatively topical or intralesional corticosteroids may improve the situation.

118.
a. This is most likely to be a Kaposi's sarcoma.
b. This increases the likelihood of a concurrent HIV infection.
c. This lesion can be treated by radiotherapy, systemic chemotherapy or intralesional chemotherapy.

119.
a. Sublingual varices.
b. Simple reassurance.

120.
a. Vitamin B_{12} deficiency is associated with a macrocytic normochromic anaemia evidenced by an increase in the mean corpuscular volume.
b. The most likely cause of vitamin B_{12} deficiency would be pernicious anaemia or intestinal malabsorption, e.g. Crohn's disease. Strict vegetarianism can also lead to B_{12} deficiency.
c. In the first instance, a Schilling test should be carried out to exclude the diagnosis of pernicious anaemia. If this proved normal, malabsorption studies would be justified.

121.
a. Clinically, this patient has pyostomatitis vegetans.
b. Histology reveals intra-epithelial microabscess formation.
c. Successful management of the patient's ulcerative colitis usually causes an improvement in the oral symptoms.

122.
a. This patient has an oral condyloma.
b. These lesions are more commonly seen in immunosuppressed individuals.
c. This lesion can be treated simply by surgical excision, although cryosurgery may also be successful.

123.
a. The majority of angular cheilitis lesions are due to *Candida*, but *Staphylococcus* and *Streptococcus*, alone or in combination, may also contribute to the clinical appearance.
b. Patients with intransigent angular cheilitis should be screened to exclude diabetes and nutritional deficiencies.

124.
a. This patient has an hereditary keratosis.
b. This can be confirmed histologically.
c. The epithelium is hyperparakeratinised and shows oedema and vacuolation.

125.
a. This patient should be asked if she has genital ulceration, since the history suggests that she may have Behçet syndrome.
b. Eye involvement would be likely in a patient with Behçet syndrome if they are HLA type A5.
c. In the original description of Behçet syndrome, anterior uveitis was the eye problem, although retinitis is more common.

126.
a. The patient may develop intra-oral bullae formation with mild trauma such as placement of a cotton wool roll. These lesions may be slow to heal and cause significant scarring.
b. Extreme gentleness and care are required when carrying out routine dental treatment.

127.
a. Cross-infection procedures should always be maintained at a standard appropriate for the care of an HIV-seropositive patient, and therefore no additional precautions are required.
b. Antibiotic prophylaxis per se is not required in order to carry out periodontal therapy in this individual. He may, however, already be taking concurrent antibiotics. Antibiotic therapy should be responsive rather than prophylactic.
c. Intense oral hygiene therapy may be necessary to bring the periodontal condition under control.

128.
a. This patient has a fissured tongue.
b. This is an innocuous and incidental finding, but a lobulated or fissured tongue may also be seen in association with geographic tongue.
c. This condition is likely to remain unchanged and asymptomatic indefinitely.

129.
a. This patient has plasma cell (allergic) gingivitis.
b. This is most likely to be a response to a topical allergen such as may be contained in toothpaste.
c. The immediate treatment for this patient is to withdraw putative allergens (e.g. toothpaste).
d. If this fails to resolve the problem, topical corticosteroid therapy, in the form of a spray, mouthwash or occlusive therapy under a veneer or splint, is warranted.

130.
a. This patient has bullous lichen planus.
b. Intense liquefactive degeneration of the basal cell layer allows bulla formation.

131.
a. Clinically, this patient has leukoplakia.
b. In this patient's case, because of the circumscribed nature of the white patch, excision biopsy is the treatment of choice.
c. This patient should be reviewed 3- to 6-monthly to monitor progress of the oral mucosa.

132.
a. This clinically is a simple amalgam tattoo, but the lesion should be radiographed and, if this is non-contributory, biopsied to reassure the patient.
b. Over 70% of cases affect the maxilla and, most commonly, the palate (47%) or gingivae (26%).

133.
a. Herpes labialis or 'cold sore'.
b. Severe, prolonged or widespread lesions may indicate underlying immunosuppression such as HIV or leukaemia, which would merit further investigation.

134.
a. Fibro-epithelial polyp—a simple fibrous nodule.
b. The patient has been using the tip of his tongue to hold the denture in place, leading to chronic irritation at this site.

135.
a. Herpes zoster or 'shingles' affecting the mandibular division of the trigeminal nerve.
b. Treatment consists of analgesia and bed rest. Systemic aciclovir is important since this has been shown to reduce the incidence of post-herpetic neuralgia.

136.
a. The history of rapid growth is suggestive of an inflammatory lesion such as pyogenic granuloma. However, differential diagnosis would include squamous cell carcinoma, Kaposi's sarcoma and syphilitic chancre.
b. The histological features of a pyogenic granuloma are loose, oedematous, moderately cellular collagenous stroma with numerous thin-walled blood vessels. The overlying epithelium is frequently ulcerated.
c. Management would consist of excision biopsy for histological assessment and reassurance of the patient. In view of the fact that the lesion is traumatic in origin, any local irritants, such as sharp cusps or denture flanges, should be removed.

137.
a. The most likely diagnosis is squamous cell carcinoma.
b. Involvement of the inferior dental nerve due to intra-osseous spread of the tumour.

138.
a. Erythema multiforme.
b. The likely precipitant is *Mycoplasma pneumoniae* (the cause of her respiratory tract infection).

139.
a. A number of topical medications might benefit the patient. Chlorhexidine 0.2% mouthwash is worth trying. Tetracycline mouthwashes are of use in some patients. A suggested regime is one 250 mg capsule to be broken open and the resultant powder dissolved in water and used as a rinse for 1 minute, without swallowing, four times daily for 1 month. Topical corticosteroids are often useful, including 0.1% triamcinolone acetonide in orabase paste, beclomethasone dipropionate spray and betamethasone 0.5 mg tablets as a mouthwash.

140.
a. It is most likely to be Crohn's disease.
b. Cobblestoning arises due to intercellular oedema aggravated by granulomata blocking lymphatic drainage.

141.
a. A vesiculobullous disorder such as mucous membrane pemphigoid.
b. Other possible oral manifestations are ulcers following rupture of the bullae (which may heal with scarring) and 'desquamative gingivitis'.
c. Treatment options will include removal of sources of oral trauma, topical corticosteroids and immune-modulating drugs such as dapsone.

142.
a. Lichen planus.
b. The variants of lichen planus encountered in the oral cavity are reticular, erosive, plaque, atrophic, papular, bullous and 'desquamative gingivitis'.

143.
a. Pseudomembranous candidosis.
b. Predisposing systemic factors are smoking, diabetes mellitus, immunosuppression (e.g. HIV, leukaemias, lymphomas), corticosteroid therapy, antibiotics and xerostomia.
c. The most likely local cause is topical or inhaled corticosteroid therapy, e.g. for use in asthma.

144.
a. There is no obvious clinical abnormality and so she may have an oral dysaesthesia or 'burning mouth syndrome'.
b. Investigations should include blood tests for full blood count, and for ferritin, folate and vitamin B_{12} levels; blood glucose; salivary flow rates; and oral microbiological sampling (especially oral rinse). Evidence of dental wear facets and parafunctional activity should be sought.
c. While the above investigations are ongoing, the patient should undergo an assessment of her psychological state, with particular reference to anxiety and depression. Any degree of cancerphobia should be explored and reassured. Her husband's death as a possible trigger should be identified and the possibility of psychiatric help or antidepressant therapy discussed openly.

145.
a. Lip-biting.
b. Reassurance, systemic analgesic drugs and antibiotic therapy—metronidazole was used in this case since the malodour was indicative of anaerobic infection.

146.
a. This is likely to have been caused by cheek-biting, secondary to a bruxist habit.
b. The patient should be reassured as to the cause of her mucosal condition and her likely life-stressors highlighted. Other evidence of myofascial pain dysfunction syndrome should be sought, e.g. muscle pain, headaches, wear facets on teeth. A simple soft occlusal splint may be helpful as a 'shock-absorber' and habit-breaker. Otherwise, appropriate physiotherapy, antidepressant or anxiolytic medication, or psychiatric referral might be of benefit, depending on the degree of symptoms and/or underlying psychological status.

147.
a. He clearly has multiple haemangiomas, which may be simple or part of a greater syndrome such as Maffucci's syndrome.
b. The patient should be examined appropriately for evidence of a medical syndrome. The lesions are best left alone unless

trauma and bleeding are problematic. The haemangiomas may be kept under observation or subjected to cryosurgery or laser therapy.

148.
a. The clinical diagnosis is speckled leukoplakia.
b. The main factors implicated in the aetiology are tobacco-smoking and alcohol consumption.
c. The patient should have a baseline incisional biopsy performed. Depending on the degree of dysplasia found, the lesion may be excised or kept under regular clinical and histological review. Advice should be given on cessation of smoking and, if relevant, reduction in alcohol consumption.

149.
a. This is simple racial pigmentation and the patient should be reassured accordingly.

150.
a. Coeliac disease, Crohn's disease and ulcerative colitis.
b. Behçet disease, cyclic neutropenia and HIV infection.

151.
a. Denture-induced hyperplasia.
b. Chronic irritation from an ill-fitting denture, with reactive tissue growth locally.
c. Removal of the denture will result in significant improvement. Then the lesion may be left or excised, according to the patient's wishes. Certainly, if new dentures are requested, the excess tissue should be removed and properly fitting dentures will prevent a recurrence of the problem.

152.
a. Sclerodactyly.
b. Secondary Sjögren's syndrome.

153.
a. Pleomorphic salivary adenoma (PSA).
b. The lesion should be biopsied, either by planned excision with a wide margin under theatre conditions, or by incision leaving sufficient tissue intra-orally to allow identification of the site if further surgery is required.
c. Histological features of a PSA include a capsule (which may be incomplete) and varied epithelial components, i.e. sheets or strands of cuboidal, columnar and myoepithelial cells; the stroma is mucoid or myxochondroid tissue and areas of cartilage may be present.

154.
a. Torus mandibularis.
b. Reassurance and leave alone.
c. The greatest difficulties would occur if the patient required a lower denture in the future, since even prosthodontists would have difficulties with these undercuts!

155.
a. Differential diagnoses to be considered are orofacial granulomatosis, Melkersson–Rosenthal syndrome, cheilitis granulomatosa and Crohn's disease.

156.
a. This is ankyloglossia or 'tongue-tie'.
b. Unless it is causing genuine problems with oral hygiene measures or dental spacing, it can be left alone; otherwise, surgical excision may be arranged.

157.
a. Stone at the parotid duct orifice.
b. Given the likely accessibility of this stone, immediate removal is indicated.

158.
a. The likely diagnosis is Sturge–Weber syndrome, with a maxillofacial haemangioma and calcification of the ipsilateral leptomeninges.
b. There is gingival enlargement secondary to phenytoin therapy.
c. There is a real risk of substantial haemorrhage following dental injection, extraction or surgery to areas of the jaws and soft tissues affected by the haemangioma. The lesions may be cavernous and deeply sited in bone.

159.
a. Median rhomboid glossitis.
b. This is a localised erythematous candidosis mainly seen in patients who smoke. Management includes an extended course of topical or systemic antifungal agents, encouragement to stop smoking and denture hygiene advice where appropriate. Patients require reassurance that this is an entirely innocuous lesion, since many are cancerphobic.

160.
a. This is desquamative gingivitis.
b. Desquamation can be reduced by gentle brushing techniques and adjuvant chlorhexidine mouthwashes.

161.
a. A stone in the submandibular duct (submandibular sialolithiasis).
b. The patient should be prescribed analgesic medication and an antibiotic such as amoxycillin. If the stone is readily palpable, it may be removed via an incision along the submandibular duct following placement of a 'holding suture' to prevent proximal movement of the stone.
c. Sialographic assessment of the gland and duct is required after the acute episode has settled. Further episodes of sialadenitis may be managed as above. Attempts to remove the stone by duct dilatation, surgery or dissolution may be successful. Frequent episodes of infection, a resultant non-functioning gland or a stone(s) in the gland itself may necessitate gland removal.

162. a. This is a technetium (radioisotope) scan or scintigraphy to investigate salivary gland function.
  b. Any autoimmune disease can be part of Sjögren's syndrome, particularly rheumatoid arthritis, systemic lupus erythematosus and primary biliary cirrhosis.
  c. Serological markers in Sjögren's syndrome include rheumatoid factor and antinuclear factor.

163. a. Given the history, antimalarial prophylactic medication is the likely cause of this area of melanosis.
  b. Other drugs implicated include phenothiazines and oral contraceptives.

164. a. This is a temporomandibular joint arthrogram which shows evidence of a fixed anterior dislocation of the intra-articular disc.
  b. The main question is whether the jaw ever locks open or closed.

165. a. The exclusion of demyelinating lesions (multiple sclerosis) and cerebellopontine angle tumours (e.g. acoustic neuromas) is important.
  b. The pain is lancinating and electric shock-like, and transfixes the patient to the spot. There may be associated lacrimation.
  c. The anti-epileptic drugs form the mainstay of treatment for trigeminal neuralgia. Carbamazepine is the first-line drug of choice, followed by phenytoin.

166. a. This is herpetiform aphthous stomatitis.
  b. This variant of aphthae is said to respond well to topical tetracycline mouthwash therapy.

167. a. This appearance points towards a vesiculobullous disorder.
  b. Special tests carried out in this patient included a blood test for indirect immunofluorescence and mucosal biopsy of an intact bulla for histological assessment and direct immunofluorescence.

168. a. This is most likely to be a lichenoid drug eruption.
  b. A mucosal biopsy would be helpful in the diagnosis.
  c. The time-scale makes the new drug therapy (e.g. diuretic or beta-blocker) a likely contender as the aetiological agent. Discussions with the patient's physician may make it possible to change to a structurally unrelated drug. However, there is, surprisingly, no guarantee that the lesions will resolve speedily or indeed at all. The patient may be managed with topical corticosteroids.

169. a. The most common drug groups involved are non-steroidal anti-inflammatories, diuretics, oral hypoglycaemics and antihypertensives (especially beta-blockers).

170.
a. Differential diagnoses would include a non-healing socket, non-Hodgkin's lymphoma and Kaposi's sarcoma.
b. The lesion should be biopsied. This proved to be a non-Hodgkin's lymphoma.

171.
a. Angular cheilitis.
b. *Candida* or *Staphylococcus* spp.
c. Swabs and smears from the lesions may be required. In addition, swabs from the anterior nares may be taken, as this site is a likely source of any *Staphylococcus*. If upper dentures are worn, swabs and smears from the fitting surface of the prosthesis and the palate are appropriate, since the denture may be the reservoir for any *Candida*.

172.
a. Ulcerative (necrotising) periodontitis.
b. The lower anterior region is most commonly affected.

173.
a. Mumps.
b. The patient should be instructed on bed rest and copious oral fluids and should be prescribed potent analgesic medication.

174.
a. This is a torus palatinus.
b. No treatment is required. Occasionally, clinical presentation makes differentiation from, for example, minor salivary gland tumours difficult, and radiographic assessment with or without biopsy may be indicated.

175.
a. Wegener's granulomatosis.
b. Cyclophosphamide therapy.

176.
a. Systemic agents available to treat severe lichen planus include prednisolone, azathioprine and retinoids.
b. Systemic corticosteroid therapy's potential side-effects are myriad and include skin striae, acne, hirsutism, hypertension, diabetes mellitus, psychiatric disturbance, osteoporosis and abnormal fat distribution.

177.
a. Malignant melanoma.
b. Metastatic melanoma carries an extremely poor prognosis.

178.
a. This patient has buccal ulceration, with bleeding and localised plaque deposits.
b. This is radiation-induced mucositis.
c. Treatment for this condition is notoriously poor but includes topical anaesthetic agents and mouthwashes such as benzydamine hydrochloride.

179.
a. Furred or coated tongue.
b. The patient's recent antibiotics may have altered his oral flora

with overgrowth of *Candida* spp. The tongue should be swabbed for culture and the patient treated according to the results. In the interim, gentle brushing of the tongue dorsum with a soft toothbrush may be helpful.

180.
a. Necrotising sialometaplasia.
b. The aetiology is largely unconfirmed, but it is thought to be an infarctive process, more common in middle-aged men who are smokers.
c. It may be confused histologically with a carcinoma, but the rapidity of clinical onset points away from this.

181.
a. Oral candidosis in a young patient would certainly raise suspicions of immunosuppression and he should be counselled appropriately in a designated centre prior to testing for HIV infection. However, the other causes of oral candidosis should not be forgotten and the patient must have a full medical work-up to include full blood count and blood glucose assays. His oral candidosis will respond to topical or systemic anti-candidal medication.
b. This patient should be encouraged to attend a sympathetic and non-judgmental dentist to discuss ongoing oral and dental care as part of a holistic approach to his management.

182.
a. This is a Kaposi's sarcoma.
b. It is thought to result from co-infection with human herpes virus type 8.

183.
a. Post-herpetic neuralgia.
b. Systemic analgesic drugs are generally unhelpful. Antidepressant drugs, anti-epileptic drugs or transcutaneous electrical nerve stimulation may prove useful. Spontaneous improvement can occur 12–18 months after onset of the pain.

184.
a. This is a hairy leukoplakia.
b. No active treatment is required. Regression may occur with systemic aciclovir and antifungal medication as treatment for Epstein–Barr virus and *Candida* spp., respectively. However, the lesion will recur on cessation of therapy.

185.
a. Many drugs can cause dryness of the oral mucosa, including antidepressants, phenothiazines and diuretics.
b. Where the medical reason for using the drug outweighs the symptoms of troublesome dry mouth, salivary substitutes may be prescribed. In addition, patients often benefit from sipping cold water or chewing sugar-free gum.

186.
a. Allergy to dietary substances such as benzoic acid and cinnamon can be identified in the majority of patients with orofacial granulomatosis by patch testing.

187.
a. Erosion of the palatal aspects of her maxillary dentition, with erythema of the palatal mucosa.
b. Induced vomiting due to bulimia nervosa.
c. Dental treatment options include composite build-ups, gold-shell crowns and topical fluoride treatment for dentine sensitivity.

188.
a. Addison's disease.
b. Measuring the blood pressure, which would be low.
c. Electrolyte measurements would show hyperkalaemia and hyponatraemia. Serum cortisol may be low. The definitive test is a synthetic ACTH stimulation test.

189.
a. This is a hyperplastic candidosis—the so-called candidal leukoplakia.
b. This is a premalignant condition and a baseline biopsy should be obtained at presentation for diagnosis and to ascertain the degree of dysplasia.

190.
a. Herpes zoster infection or 'shingles'.
b. The infection occurs within the distribution of a dermatome and is therefore inevitably unilateral.

191.
a. Black hairy tongue.
b. Poor oral hygiene and lack of a normal 'rough' diet allow overgrowth of keratin on the tongue dorsum. This keratin layer is subsequently invaded by chromogenic bacteria and stained with cigarette smoke and dietary pigments (tannins) to give the appearance shown.

192.
a. Fordyce granules or spots—simple sebaceous glands.
b. Fifty per cent of the population have some intra-oral sebaceous glands, but these are seldom so prominent.

193.
a. Psoriasis.
b. Geographic tongue.

194.
a. Pleomorphic salivary adenoma, monomorphic salivary adenoma and adenolymphoma.
b. Adenoid cystic carcinoma, which tends to spread perineurally.

195.
a. The patient also has chronic erythematous candidosis of the hard palate—the reservoir for *Candida* organisms implicated in angular cheilitis.

b. In addition to microbiological sampling from the lips, nares, denture and palate, haematological investigations (full blood count, ferritin, vitamin B_{12}, folate and blood glucose) are warranted.

c. Topical treatments will be determined by the results of microbiological sampling, but a good generic medication is miconazole cream which has activity against *Staphylococcus* and *Candida* organisms. Any evidence of reservoirs in the nares or mouth should be dealt with using appropriate topical agents, denture hygiene and, where necessary, systemic antimicrobial therapy.

196.
a. This is a lichenoid eruption, possibly related to the amalgam restoration.
b. Patch testing should be carried out if available. Removal of the amalgam is likely to cause clinical improvement in any event.

197.
a. It is a soft full-coverage occlusal splint.
b. MPDS is classically a constant, dull pre-auricular or auricular pain which may be unilateral or bilateral. There may be acute exacerbations of pain, with sharp, shooting radiations. There may be trismus, audible clicks on jaw movement, joint tenderness, tenderness in the muscles of mastication and associated headaches.
c. Other treatments include physiotherapy and antidepressant drugs.

198.
a. Systemic lupus erythematosus
b. Oral lesions are best managed with topical corticosteroids applied as a mouthwash, paste or spray. They may also respond to the systemic medication prescribed for the condition generally, e.g. prednisolone or azathioprine.

199.
a. Tuberculosis or lymphoma.
b. The patient should be referred to a general physician.

200.
a. During the luteal phase premenstrually.
b. Pregnancy causes temporary remission in 80% of female sufferers.

201.
a. Desquamative gingivitis.
b. Direct and indirect immunofluorescence.

202.
a. Vesiculobullous disorders.
b. Investigations should include oral mucosal biopsy for direct immunofluorescence and a blood sample for indirect immunofluorescence.
c. The eyes should be examined for conjunctival scarring by an

ophthalmologist and the nasal mucosa by an otorhinolaryngologist, if there is any suggestion of nasal bleeding or discharge.

203.
a. Non-migratory geographic tongue (erythema migrans perstans).
b. Reassurance is all that is required.

204.
a. The patient should be encouraged to stop any risk factors, such as smoking and heavy alcohol consumption. Any underlying nutritional deficiency and chronic candidal infection should be excluded. Any contributing intra-oral trauma should be removed. In view of the risk of malignant transformation, the lesion should be excised.
b. This patient should have regular follow-up appointments, with subsequent mucosal biopsies. Encouragement to stop smoking and alcohol consumption should be reiterated at each visit.

205.
a. This ulcer is a non-specific ulcer, related to HIV disease. It does not have the classical features of an aphthous ulcer.
b. The ulcer should be biopsied and assessed for viruses such as CMV, bacteria such as *Mycobacterium*, and fungi such as *Candida* spp. If no clear infective aetiological agent is established, the ulcer may respond to topical or intralesional corticosteroids or systemic corticosteroid medication. However, these ulcers can be very difficult to eradicate.

206.
a. This is chemical burn damage due to aspirin being placed adjacent to the painful tooth.
b. The toothache should be relieved and the tongue left to heal without intervention. The patient should be reviewed to ensure adequate healing.

207.
a. This is nicotinic stomatitis.
b. These are the duct orifices of minor salivary glands.

208.
a. This is likely to be a hairy leukoplakia.
b. Frictional keratosis and smoker's keratosis.

209.
a. This is a sublingual keratosis.
b. This lesion should be biopsied to determine the presence and degree of dysplasia. Further treatment depends on the result of this special test.
c. The risk of malignant transformation is higher in sublingual lesions.

210.
a. Athlete's foot.
b. No. This is due to a dermatophyte infection which is quite different from candidosis.

c. Polyene antifungal agents (e.g. nystatin) are ineffective against dermatophytes. Miconazole (an imidazole) cream is, however, effective.

211.
a. This is a wart.
b. Human papilloma virus (HPV).
c. Molecular biological techniques, such as in situ hybridisation or the polymerase chain reaction, may be used to demonstrate HPV DNA in the tissues.

212.
a. This is likely to be a Kaposi's sarcoma.
b. Sixty per cent of Kaposi's sarcomas occur in the head and neck region; the palate is the most common intra-oral site.

213.
a. This is Peutz–Jeghers syndrome.
b. Hamartomatous polyps are found in the stomach, small intestine and colon.
c. This exhibits an autosomal dominant inheritance pattern.

214.
a. This is stomatitis gangrenosum.
b. Other types of oral ulceration in inflammatory bowel disease include recurrent aphthous stomatitis and pyostomatitis vegetans.

215.
a. The radiological assessment reveals no abnormality and the diagnosis is atypical facial pain.
b. The patient should undergo a full assessment to exclude dental and sinus pathology. A full psychosocial assessment is warranted, with the likely outcome of psychotherapy or antidepressant medication.

Index